Lectures on Yoga

Lectures on Yoga

Practical Lessons on Yoga

by Swami Rama

Published by
The Himalayan International Institute
of Yoga Science and Philosophy
Honesdale, Pennsylvania

Library of Congress Catalog Card Number: 76-359603

ISBN 0-89389-050-2 (cloth)
ISBN 0-89389-051-0 (paper)

© 1979 by
The Himalayan International Institute of Yoga
Science and Philosophy of the U.S.A.
RD 1, Box 88
Honesdale, Pennsylvania 18431

Sixth Edition 1979
2nd Printing 1983

Printed in U.S.A.

Contents

Preface

There are seven schools of Indian philosophy, ranging from the materialistic point of view to its diametric opposite in which matter is considered to be a mere shadow of the spirit. The Sankhya and Yoga schools of philosophy take a point midway between these two extremes. They came into existence gradually, after a long period of growth and experimentation, and they are complementary. Yoga deals with the experiential aspects of man's liberation from human imperfection and suffering, and is concerned with practical methods for attaining this state, using the philosophical doctrines of Sankhya as their basis.

The Sankhya school of philosophy, founded by the sage, Kapila, around 600 B.C., admits of two ultimate realities: *purusha* or cosmic consciousness and *prakrti* or elemental matter. The manifest universe evolves out of *prakrti*; it results from the coming together of *purusha* and *prakrti*, matter being permeated by consciousness. What is more, this scheme of evolution applies both to the macrocosm—the universe, and to the microcosm—man. Yoga bases its teachings on this scheme of evolution in man—the microcosm; it concerns itself with the practical aspects of involution, or the return from identification with the manifest body and mind to ultimate consciousness.

The main teaching of yoga is that man's true nature is divine, but that he is unaware of his true nature and therefore falsely identifies with his body and his intellect— both of which are within *prakriti*, or matter, and hence subject to decay and death. All of man's misery is, therefore, a consequence of this false identification. Yoga leads one to realization of the Self, and with such realization comes liberation from all human imperfections.

There are many paths to realization of the Self, just as there are many spokes from the rim of a wheel to its center, and yoga is used in a generic sense for all of these different paths. Some of them are:

Karma yoga	The yoga of action
Bhakti yoga	The yoga of devotion
Jnana yoga	The yoga of knowledge
Kundalini yoga	The yoga of awakening latent power
Raja yoga	The royal path

The teachings of raja yoga, which is the subject of this book, encompass the teachings of all the different paths; it concerns itself with three dimensions, or realms— the physical, the mental and the spiritual. Through the methods of raja yoga one achieves mastery of all three realms and is thus led to full realization of the Self.

The teachings of raja yoga go back many thousands of years, and little is known of their beginnings, but they are considered to be revealed teachings of divine origin. Somewhere around 200 B.C., they were systematized and codified by the sage, Patanjali, who organized the teachings into 196 *sutras*, or aphorisms, the *Yoga Sutras* of Patanjali which consist of four *padas* or chapters. The first deals with *samadhi*—the state of self-realization, the second with the practical means towards this end, the third with the powers that manifest themselves in one who treads the path of yoga, while the last chapter deals with *kaivalya*, or liberation.

Raja yoga, also known as *astanga* yoga, or the eight-fold path, outlines the practical means of achieving the state of self-realization. It is made up of eight *angas* or limbs: *yama, niyama, asana, pranayama, pratyahara, dharana, dhyana* and *samadhi*; the first five limbs are called the external limbs, the last three are internal. The *yamas* and *niyamas* constitute the moral code of yoga and help one to cultivate the right mental attitudes. *Asana*, or posture, aims at physical well-being and control over the body, for a healthy body is a prerequisite for a healthy and controlled mind. *Pranayama* is control of *prana*, or the life force, achieved through control of the most gross manifestation of *prana*—the breath. One can control the mind only if one can control one's breathing. *Pratyahara* is withdrawal of the senses and is necessary if one is to achieve tranquility of mind.

The internal limbs focus more directly on control of the mind. *Dharana* is attention and concentration; it helps to bring the diffuse mind to a point of focus. Prolonged *dharana* leads to a state of *dhyana*, or meditation, characterized by one-pointedness of the mind, while prolonged *dhyana* leads to *samadhi*, the state of self-realization. Here, the mind is transcended, and one becomes aware of the Self and is united with it. This state is characterized by *sat-chit-ananda*, or existence, consciousness and bliss. One expands one's consciousness, and becomes one with the ultimate reality.

Raja yoga is, therefore, a systematic and scientific discipline that leads one to ultimate truth. Most religions teach one what to do; raja yoga teaches one how to be. Unlike religions, it does not impose unquestioning faith but encourages healthy discrimination. It leads finally to liberation.

By following the path prescribed one can verify for oneself its central hypothesis that man's true nature is divine. It is, therefore, not only an ancient, esoteric Eastern philosophy, but it is also a practical, systematic and scientific quest for the infinite, relevant and necessary in the modern context both in the East and in the West. If incorporated into modern education raja yoga would equip one to deal with the conflicts, frustrations and turmoil inevitable in all modern societies. Through it, man can realize his fullest potential for creative thought and action. Furthermore through raja yoga he can transcend all human limitations and realize his true nature.

ONE

What is Yoga?

The word *yoga* is much used and much misunderstood these days, for our present age is one of faddism, and yoga has often been reduced to the status of a fad. Many false and incomplete teachings have been propagated in its name, it has been subject to commercial exploitation, and one small aspect of yoga is often taken to be all of yoga. For instance, many people in the West think it is a physical and beauty cult, while others think it is a religion. All of this has obscured the real meaning of yoga. Let me try to give you a glimpse of its true nature.

Yoga is a systematic science; its teachings are an integral part of most religions, but yoga itself is not a religion. Most religions teach one what to do, but yoga teaches one how to be. Yoga practices, however, described in symbolic language, may be found in the sacred scriptures of most religions. The book of Genesis and the book of Revelations contain such teachings, and in the book of Psalms there are many references to yogic methods of meditation. Psalm 119:15, 23, 48, 78, 97 and 148, for instance, mentions meditation frequently. There is also considerable similarity between the underlying philosophy upon which yoga is based (*Sankhya* philosophy) and the teachings found in Judaism. Aspects of the yogic science of breath, for instance, can be found in the kaballah where the link between breath and spirit has always been acknowledged.

In the Christian tradition Saint Francis of Assisi was one of the greatest yogis that the West has produced. Saint Bernard, Saint Ignatius, Saint Teresa, Saint John of the Cross, Dionysius and Meister Eckhart were also great Christian yogis. Mystics of all religions of the world have practiced yoga in one form or another. However, with the passage of time the symbolic language in which these teachings were veiled has been misinterpreted, so that much of the original teaching has been lost or distorted into meaningless ritualism. But these same teachings are alive within the tradition of yoga even today. Yoga is not an ancient, esoteric Eastern philosophy; it is a practical, systematic and scientific quest for perfection, as relevant today as it was in ancient times, as relevant in the West as in the East.

The origins of yoga are obscure; they go back many thousands of years and are considered to be divine rather than human. India is a stronghold of this science because the original purity of the teachings has been maintained there—because yoga teachings have been handed down in India through a living tradition, the master-discipleship tradition. Yoga teachings were systematized by a sage named Patanjali who, around 200 B.C., codified the teachings into 196 short aphorisms, or *sutras*. There are several manuals and manuscripts, not yet translated into English or any other modern language, which help in understanding and practicing the aphorisms of Patanjali, but there are also well-known commentaries on the *sutras*, such as those of Vyasa-Bhashya and Vachaspati-Misra.

The central teaching of yoga is that man's true nature is divine, perfect and infinite. He is unaware of this divinity, however, because he falsely identifies himself with his body, mind and objects of the external world. This false identification, in turn, makes him think he is imperfect and limited, subject to sorrow, decay and death because his mind and body are subject to the limitations of time, space and causation. Through the meditative methods of yoga, however, man can cast off this ignorance and become aware of his own true Self which is pure and free from all imperfections. The Sanskrit word *yoga* comes from the root *yuj*, meaning to join together, or unite, and yoga represents the union of the individual self, or *atman*, with the supreme universal Self, or *Paramatman*. This is the union of man with absolute reality. The same concept is described in the Bible by the word *yoke*, meaning mystic union.

The modern age is a machine age, most modern societies are obsessed by power, and much time and effort are wasted in trying to discover more powerful and more destructive weapons. Technology has made rapid progress, but man has not. He has learned to harness atomic energy, but is unable to control his own senses and his own mind. The danger of atomic weapons lies not in the powerful destructive devices themselves; it arises because of the uncontrolled minds of the men who are corrupted by their power.

All of man's efforts have been directed outwards, and little evolution has taken place in his inner world. His instincts, urges, passions, emotions, thoughts and actions are as primitive today as they were in less advanced ages. He is engrossed in ignorance which is characterized by restlessness, a blind clinging to earthly existence, perverted individualism, voluptuous abandonment to sensual pleasures, violence, strife and discord.

Man, in his ignorance, chases the fleeting shadows of wealth, position and power, but he can derive no real happiness from finite objects that are conditioned by time, space and causation. His wants are insatiable, and he is always dissatisfied. One dollar of pleasure is mixed with ninety-nine dollars of pain, fear and worry. True happiness, inner peace and contentment elude him. In affluent societies there are many men who have satisfied their basic needs, who have many comforts and luxuries as well as sizeable savings, men who have achieved prestige and a position of power in their professions, who have healthy and intelligent families—yet they are discontent and searching. In spite of everything they have, there is still something lacking in their lives, and so they continue to search for it in the outside world. Little do they realize that what they lack is inner peace which the world outside can never give them. Few truly realize that happiness is a state of mind, that amidst the din and boisterous bustle of worldly activities there appear moments of tranquility and peace when the mind soars above temporary pleasures and reflects on the higher mysteries of life. In these moments every man is a philosopher. He then begins to search for the truth, and discrimination dawns on him. If such a man adopts the meditative life, even amidst his worldly activities, he will eventually attain the highest wisdom and the highest bliss of self-realization.

The whole process of yoga is an ascent into the purity of that absolute perfection which is the original state of man. It implies, therefore, the removal of enveloping impurities, the stilling of lower feelings and thoughts and the establishment of a state of perfect balance and harmony. All the methods of yoga have ethical and moral perfection as their basis, and thus a new world order of love could easily be effected by the adoption of even the simplest and most fundamental observances of yogic discipline.

The greatest problem for the beginner is his inherent restlessness of mind. Mind, by its very nature, is ever outgoing and unsteady. The highest state of meditation, however, requires a one-pointed mind, free from attachments and worldly desires. This is why attachment of the mind towards worldly objects is the arch enemy of the student of yoga. To reach subtler levels of consciousness one needs will power, discrimination, firm control of the mind as well as conscious direction of its powers towards the desired end, and this is possible only through a resolute turning away from worldly attachments, a determined effacement of the ego, a deliberate stoppage of all inharmonious mental processes and a constant dwelling upon the ultimate goal. To achieve this one need not renounce home and society and retire to the solitude of a mountain cave. One can achieve a state of non-attachment and desirelessness at home, while engaging in worldly activities, if yogic discipline becomes a part of one's daily life. True renunciation of worldly desires is a mental state; it does not necessarily need to be a physical act of renunciation. But success is possible only with constant and intense practice, always keeping in mind that the ultimate aim is perfection and bliss.

There are four stages of non-attachment:

1. The first stage is to make a sincere attempt at not allowing the mind to dwell on sensual objects.

2. When objects attract the student, he should endeavor to free himself from those attractions. When discrimination dawns gradually, non-attachment develops and equilibrium is established.

3. Even after the senses have been subdued the mind still has hatred and affection for worldly objects because the mind can function independently of the senses.

4. In the higher stages of non-attachment the objects of the world do not tempt one at all. The senses are under control, and the mind is perfectly free from likes and dislikes and all other pairs of opposites. The aspirant has now gained independence and supremacy. Without non-attachment, no spiritual progress is possible.

Let us now consider the prerequisites for one who decides to tread the path of yoga towards spiritual enlightenment. Good health, a sound mind, sincerity and a burning desire for liberation from human imperfections are necessary prerequisites. Good health is ensured by a simple and well regulated diet, adequate sleep, some physical exercise and relaxation. Purity of food leads to purity of mind. Heavy food leads to inertia. Milk, fruits, fresh vegetables, nuts and the like are helpful if they are in proper balance. One also needs a suitable place for the practice of yoga exercises and meditation. It should be maintained at a moderate temperature throughout the year and should be well-ventilated, free from dampness, clean and quiet. In addition, since all distractions, disturbances and diseases arise from an imbalance of the three *doshas*—wind, bile and phlegm (too much phlegm, for instance, makes the body heavy, inert and stiff), one should choose one's diet and the place for practice so as to maintain a balance of these three.

Yoga science has two aspects—theoretical and practical. Theory can be learned through books and scriptures but a perfect guide, or *guru*, is needed for the practical aspect. The word *guru* means, "one who dispels the darkness of ignorance," and he is needed because in yoga there are several different methods that work towards the same goal of perfection. Only a *guru* can select and prescribe one that is suitable to the upbringing, circumstances, mind and nature of the student. One who tries to learn the practical aspect of yoga through books or from attending a few lectures, is often bewildered by the great variety and diversity of techniques available in yoga. He gains nothing by trying a little of everything, and even if he is sincere, his effort is wasted. A true yogi will always lead the student systematically through the complex stages of yoga to the ultimate state of perfection.

These days there are many yogis who claim to be perfect masters, and it is hard to know how one distinguishes the true *guru* from the many imposters. But when a student prepares himself by increasing his mental capacities, he starts discriminating between right and wrong and between useful and useless values in the area of learning and teaching, and he becomes able to evaluate various teachers accordingly. The Upanishads, which are ancient yogic scriptures, state that when the disciple is ready, the master appears. This means that when a student has an intense desire for truth in his heart he will receive divine help sooner or later. Fortunate indeed is a student who has the blessings and guidance of a *guru*!

As mentioned earlier, there are many different methods of yoga, all leading to the same goal of self-realization. The methods vary so as to accommodate varying temperaments and capacities, but they are like the different spokes of a wheel; they all meet at the same center—self-realization. The different paths of yoga are not mutually exclusive; they merely represent a difference of emphasis. Let us briefly consider some of these different paths:

1. Karma yoga—The yoga of action. This path teaches one to do one's own duty skillfully and selflessly, dedicating the fruits of his actions to humanity. This yoga helps one to live successfully in the world while remaining above it, unaffected by worldly fetters.

2. Bhakti yoga—The yoga of devotion. This path is known as the path of love and devotion. It is the path of self-surrender, of devoting and

dedicating all of one's resources to attaining the ultimate reality.

3. Jnana yoga—The yoga of knowledge. This path involves intense discrimination. Knowledge dawns on one who persistently discriminates between the real and the unreal, between the transient and the everlasting, between the finite and the infinite. This path is tread by only a fortunate few who systematically contemplate the higher and subtler realities of life.

4. Kundalini yoga—This is a highly technical subject which needs the guidance of a competent teacher even though there are various manuals and methods for awakening the serpent-like vital force that remains sleeping in the city of life in every human body.

5. Mantra yoga—In the deep state of meditation the highly accomplished sages in ancient times received certain sounds which are traditionally transmitted to the student, and which are to be used as objects of concentration. There are many varieties of *mantras* which help the student in purification, concentration and meditation.

6. Hatha yoga—*Ha* and *tha* are symbolic syllables used to indicate the flow of the breath in the right and left nostrils. Hatha yoga deals mostly with body and breathing exercises which prepare the student to become aware of his internal states. Hatha yoga exercises are designed in such a way that the body becomes an instrument for

treading the path of the higher life.

7. Raja yoga—This "royal path" is highly scientific. It was systemized by the codifier of yoga, Patanjali, and by following it one learns to control his desires, emotions and thoughts as well as the subtle impressions which lie dormant in the unconscious. It unites the individual to the cosmic reality by means of the eight rungs in the yoga ladder which are systematically explained and described. The aspirant finally attains the eighth rung, called *samadhi*.

As emphasized earlier, these paths are not mutually exclusive. Every student of yoga practices them all to some extent, for perfection comes only when man develops his actions, speech and mind together. One-sided development is not desirable. Karma yoga helps one to perform his duties in the external world so that his actions become means rather than obstacles in the path of self-realization. Bhakti yoga develops devotion and faith and destroys hindrances to concentration and meditation. It makes one into a gentle being and develops a zeal for giving. In this way relations with others become harmonious. Jnana yoga removes the veil of ignorance and develops the power of discrimination and will. Study and contemplation of the scriptures, with the aid of a competent teacher, completely and finally help one in attaining self-realization. Raja yoga steadies the mind and makes it one-pointed. The differences between the different paths of yoga lie in the preliminaries to the final stages and in the methods of concentration they prescribe, but the final three stages of development are common to all. These are the stages of concentration, meditation and the final union of *samadhi*. They all lead to the state of perfection, wisdom and bliss. The yoga described by Patanjali in his *Yoga Sutras* is raja yoga, the royal path. It encompasses teachings from all the different paths, and because of the variety of methods it includes, it can be practiced by people of varying backgrounds and temperaments. Raja yoga is involved with three dimensions or realms: physical, mental and spiritual; through its methods one achieves mastery of all three and is thus led to full realization of the Self. It is a systematic and scientific discipline that does not impose unquestioning faith, but encourages healthy discrimination. Certain practices are prescribed, along with the benefits derived from them so raja yoga can, therefore, be scientifically verified by anyone who accepts its methods as a hypothesis to be tested by his own experience. Because of this, raja yoga is ideally suited to modern times in which skepticism is almost a religion.

Raja yoga is also called astanga yoga, or "the eightfold path," because its eight steps trace a systematic path of regulation and control from the gross (the physical body), to the subtler (the senses), to the subtlest manifestations of the mind. The eight steps are *yama, niyama, asana, pranayama, pratyahara, dharana, dhyana* and *samadhi*; they will be described briefly here, and in succeeding chapters they will be discussed in detail.

The first four steps—*yama, niyama, asana* and *pranayama*, comprise the path of hatha yoga which is both auxiliary and preliminary to the last four stages of raja yoga. *Yama* and *niyama* are the ten commitments of yoga of which the five *yamas*, or restraints, are non-violence, truthfulness, non-stealing, continence and non-possessive-ness. Their practice leads to behavioral modifications, in which all imperfections are replaced by virtues. The five *niyamas*, or observances, are cleanliness (both external and internal), contentment, practices which bring about perfection of body and senses (*tapas*), study of the scriptures and surrender to the ultimate reality. The *niyamas* regulate one's habits and hence lead to the control of one's behavior, for actions, when repeated, crystallize into habits, and these habits, in the course of time, are incorporated as definite traits in one's personality. The beginner should not be discouraged by the immensity of these first two steps of raja yoga. He is not asked to perfect the *yamas* and *niyamas* before proceeding further, but he should try to practice them as conscientiously as he can. With persistent effort he will eventually be able to perfect them. When hatha yoga is taught in the West, however, only *asana* and certain breathing exercises are taught. The *yamas* and *niyamas* are usually neglected because of the difficulties they entail and the changes of life style that are necessary in order to practice them. Hatha yoga has, therefore, degenerated into a cult of physical beauty and prolonged youth. *Asanas* and breathing exercises ensure physical health and harmony, it is true, but their full benefits can be realized only by one whose mind is free from violent and distracting emotions, and it is *yama* and *niyama* that enable the student to cultivate a steady and tranquil mind.

The third step in raja yoga is *asana*, or posture, of which there are two types: meditative postures and postures which ensure physical well-being. A stable, meditative posture leads, in the course of time, to a stable mind, for the mind and body interact to an amazing degree. If the body is uncomfortable and unsteady it acts upon the mind, making it unsteady and distracted. Experience has shown that a posture suitable for meditation should be comfortable and stable, ensuring that the head, neck and trunk be erect and in a straight line. Such a posture makes it possible for one to have a motionless body, thus preventing unchecked restlessness from disturbing the mind and dissipating the will. The beginner should select and cultivate one posture and not change it continually. The second kind of posture is practiced to perfect the body, making it supple and free from disease. These postures control specific muscles and nerves and hence have therapeutic benefits. For instance, yogis have cured diseases such as leprosy with the posture called *mayurasana*, the peacock posture; the yogic posture of relaxation, called *shavasana*, in conjunction with certain breathing techniques, can cure hypertension, heart ailments and several other imbalances of body and mind. Specific postures and their therapeutic effects will be studied in detail in a later chapter.

The fourth step of raja yoga is *pranayama*, or control of *prana*, the vital energy that sustains body and mind. The grossest manifestation of *prana* is the breath, so *pranayama* is also called the science of breathing. Regulation of breath leads to regulation of the mind, for if the mind is disturbed, there is a corresponding disturbance in the breathing, and vice-versa. This is easily observed in one who is afraid, excited, overcome by passion and the like. His breathing is rapid and irregular.

By the same token, continuous regulation of the breathing rhythm leads to a calm mind. In addition, the exercises of *pranayama* purify and strengthen the nervous system.

The fifth step of raja yoga is *pratyahara* or withdrawal and control of the senses. The mind contacts the objects of the world through the five senses of sight, hearing, touch, taste and smell. It is thus constantly gathering sensations from the external world, and these sensations set it to wandering. The student of yoga should therefore acquire the ability to voluntarily draw the senses inward and thus isolate himself from the distractions of the world outside. To do this the student should always be aware of the sense organs and should attempt to control their activity (this is not a physical process but a voluntary, mental one), for sense withdrawal from external objects is an essential preliminary to concentration.

Dharana, or concentration, is the sixth step in raja yoga. In concentration the dissipated powers of the mind are gathered together and directed towards the object of concentration through continued voluntary attention. Involuntary attention is effortless, but in voluntary attention a conscious effort of the will is involved which is developed through perseverance. When it is strengthened the student is able to concentrate, and then there is a focusing of the mind on the object of concentration which may be an external object or a mental concept (the *guru* usually chooses a suitable object for concentration, based on his judgment of the student's abilities and needs). Through *dharana*, or concentration, the diffused mind is focused and hence made more powerful and penetrative. Therefore, in order to fulfill the latent potentials of the mind one should systematically cultivate the ability to concentrate.

Prolonged, unbroken concentration leads to the state of meditation, or *dhyana*, which is the seventh step in raja yoga. Concentration makes the mind one-pointed and steady. Meditation expands the one-pointed mind to the superconscious state by piercing through its conscious and subconscious levels. Meditation is the uninterrupted flow of the mind towards one object or concept, and with this flow intuitive knowledge dawns. All methods of yoga prepare one to reach the stage of meditation, for only through meditation can one reach the level of the superconscious mind and hence attain perfection.

Why is meditation necessary? Just as there is a subconscious state beneath the conscious state, so is there a superconscious state above the conscious state. Meditation alone can take man to this blissful state of mind. Few people reach it because it is possible to get there only through persistent effort, and only after meditation has become a part of one's life.

Meditation can also help one to overcome physical and psychological problems. A large percentage of all diseases is psychosomatic, arising from conflicts, repressions and suppressions in the unconscious mind. Meditation leads one to an awareness of these conflicts, helps one to analyze them and then erase them, thus establishing harmony at the unconscious level.

No truly intellectual man could possibly be satisfied with modern education. It is superficial, one-sided, and it involves repetitious parroting; it does not help one to know, develop and control one's internal states. Meditation alone can help one to do this. Man then becomes aware of his latent powers and is able to control his subtler energies, thus becoming more creative and dynamic. In such a man the so-called supernatural powers of telepathy, clairvoyance and the like arise spontaneously. His limitations begin to drop away, and "miracles" are within his abilities. The prophets of all religions were, through their meditative prowess, able to perform many "miracles" which were not really miracles at all, but only the fulfilling of the natural potential within all human beings. The training and discipline needed to reach such a state, however, ensure against the misuse of these powers for selfish ends. A wise man regards such powers merely as by-products of the yogic discipline, indications of progress. His sole aim is union with the cosmic spirit, and he is not blinded by the powers. He simply continues to practice the disciplines till he reaches the state of perfection.

Prolonged and intense meditation leads to the last step of raja yoga—the state of *samadhi*, or the superconscious state. In this state man becomes one with the divine Self and transcends all imperfections and limitations. This is the state of mystic union described in Christian, Buddhist, Mohammedan and Hindu scriptures. The state of *samadhi* is also known as the fourth state of sleepless sleep which transcends the three normal states of waking, dreaming and dreamless sleep. A man who has attained *samadhi* is a blessing to society, for if humanity is to achieve a better civilization, it is possible only through the growth of the inner being. The entire life of a man who is established in *samadhi* is a spontaneous expression of the unhindered flow of supreme consciousness.

The physical sciences are based on sense perceptions that are interpreted by the rational faculty. Sense
perceptions and rationality, however, are limited by
time, space and causation. They do not give us a complete
understanding of the various forces shaping man and all
creation. Yoga science is the soul of all sciences and all
philosophies. It can solve the basic problems of modern
man, both in the East and in the West. It is definite and
systematic, and it leads one to the highest source of
knowledge which is called intuitive knowledge. The
teachings of yoga have been handed down to us because of
the ancient yogis of India who lived selfless lives, renounc-
ing worldly cares and pleasures in order to devote themselves to the meditative life. Their unique experiences
enabled them to understand and interpret correctly the
true nature of matter, mind and energy, and this
knowledge, gleaned from their intuitive experiences, was
then expressed outwardly and in a systematic manner. It
is this direct knowledge that has been handed down from
guru to disciple in a long chain from ancient times to the
present day. Fortunate indeed is the sincere aspirant who
comes into contact with this continuous and spontaneous
flow of truth! Through these ancient teachings he can
raise the capacity of his mind to perceive, assimilate and
respond to the infinite consciousness which is the basis of
all manifestation.

TWO

Yama and Niyama

The mind and body interact to a greater extent than is normally imagined. In fact, modern scientific findings are beginning to indicate that most diseases are physical manifestations of mental and emotional disturbances. In other words, physical health is dependent on mental well-being, and it is therefore necessary to cultivate mental attitudes which ensure a steady and tranquil mind before one turns his attention to physical well-being. That is why the rungs of *asana* and *pranayama* are preceded by *yama* and *niyama*—if the mind is subject to unsettling emotions, the resulting bodily disturbances cannot be combated by any of the known *asanas*. The value of *asanas* and *pranayama* is therefore limited unless they are taught in conjunction with the *yamas* and *niyamas*, the moral code, or "ten commitments," of raja yoga.

Yama

The *yamas* are the five restraints which regulate

one's relationship with other beings. They are: *ahimsa*, or non-violence; *satya*, or truthfulness; *asteya*, or non-stealing; *brahmacharya*, or abstinence from sensual indulgence; *aparigraha*, or non-possessiveness.

Ahimsa literally means non-hurting, or non-violence. One normally thinks of violence only in terms of the physical, and most people in civilized societies refrain from gross acts of physical violence. *Ahimsa*, however, refers to non-violence in thought and word as well as in deed. Violence in speech or in action is almost always preceded by violent thoughts, and violent thoughts have serious repercussions on the mind and on the body—they should be avoided, if only for this reason. On the positive side, careful cultivation of *ahimsa* leads to a spontaneous, all-encompassing love. One begins to see the unity in all creation and thus progresses towards the goal of self-realization.

Satya, or truthfulness, is an essential part of all codes of morality in all societies. One should be truthful to oneself and to others in thought, word and deed. As most people know, one lie inevitably leads to another, and soon deception becomes second nature and leads to a fearful and scheming mind. It is said that if one makes truth the central focus of his life, all of his utterances will come true, for such a one is incapable of untruth.

Asteya, or non-stealing, includes refraining from misappropriation, accepting bribes and the like. The desire for what another owns can be very strong, for the mind, when possessed by it, is capable of little else. Such an attitude of mind is based on underlying feelings of inadequacy and jealousy, a sense of having been cheated and a desire for retribution. One is haunted by the thought that "someone else has what I need in order to feel complete and fulfilled." But stealing an external object does not get rid of the basic sense of inadequacy, so one surreptitiously takes, again and again. Still, the underlying feelings remain. Cultivating *asteya* counteracts such attitudes. It helps to develop a sense of completeness and self-sufficiency and leads to freedom from the bondage of such cravings.

Brahmacharya literally means, "to walk in Brahman." One who cultivates this *yama* is therefore aware of Brahman alone. Such a state is possible only if the mind is free from all sensual desires, and of all sensual desires, the sexual urge is the most powerful and the most destructive. *Brahmacharya* is therefore often translated as abstinence from sex, or celibacy. In reality, it refers to continence in either the celibate or the married state, for sexual excesses lead to the dissipation of vital energy which could instead be used to attain deeper states of consciousness. *Brahmacharya* should not, however, be interpreted as repression of sensual urges—repression leads only to frustration and an abnormal state of mind. *Brahmacharya* means control of and freedom from all sensual cravings. The bliss that accompanies self-realization is far greater than any transient sensual pleasure, and one whose goal is self-realization would therefore overcome the obstacles of sensual cravings without any kind of suppression.

Aparigraha, or non-possessiveness, has been misunderstood to mean denying oneself all material possessions. But as is the case with each of these restraints, this practice fosters an inward attitude rather than an outward appearance. It involves not being addicted to, or dependent on, one's possessions rather than the outward denial of them. A beggar, for instance, could be more attached to his begging bowl than a king to all his treasures. The danger lies not in having material possessions; it lies in becoming attached to them or in craving more.

Niyama

The *niyamas* are the observances one should follow, and are five in number. They are: *shaucha*, or purity; *santosha*, or contentment; *tapas*, or practices that lead to perfection of body and mind and senses; *swadhyaya*, or study that leads to knowledge of the Self; *Ishwara-pra-nidhana*, or surrender to the ultimate reality.

Saucha involves purity, both of the body and the mind. Purity of the body is easily achieved, but not purity of the mind. To achieve this state one should cultivate *smriti* or mindfulness and *buddhi*, or discrimination. That is, one should always be aware of one's thoughts, and one should learn to discriminate between pure and impure thoughts on the basis of whether they lead to greater freedom or to greater bondage and ignorance. Sincerity and perseverance are essential in cultivating this *niyama*.

Santosha, or contentment, is a state of mind which is not dependent on one's material status. A beggar, for instance, can be as content as a king, if not more so. Man's desires are insatiable, and no sooner is one fulfilled than another arises. The mind is therefore in a constant state of agitation, and tranquility is possible only through the cultivation of *santosha*. But contentment should not lead to slackening of effort. Rather, effort should stem from a sense of duty and service instead of from discontent or anticipation of the fruits of one's efforts.

Tapas has often been wrongly interpreted as excessive austerity and mortification of the flesh, as exemplified by hair shirts and beds of nails. But in the Bhagavad Gita the Lord Krishna clearly states that yoga is not for him who indulges the flesh nor for him who tortures it. *Tapas* literally means, "that which generates heat," for heat arises in one who is full of spiritual fervor, one with a burning zeal for enlightenment. Acts which increase this spiritual fervor constitute *tapas*. So a simple life free from sensual indulgence, regulated fasting, chanting the name of the Lord and serving one's fellow men, all constitute *tapas*. Through *tapas* one develops strength of body and mind, and the blaze of spiritual fervor burns brighter.

Swadhyaya is study leading to knowledge of the Self. This begins with intellectual pursuits—understanding the scriptures and other books of spiritual value. Rational acceptance of spiritual truths leads, upon further reflection and meditation, to intuitive insights and then to the true understanding of these truths which is supported by study of the internal states of consciousness. Only then does knowledge of the Self begin to dawn on the aspirant.

Ishwara-pranidhana, or surrender to the ultimate reality, is possible only with infinite faith and dedication. This is total surrender and is achieved only through time, sincerity and perseverance. The ego has great tenacity and resists such complete surrender, but when it is transcended, knowledge of one's true nature is attained.

One could easily be overwhelmed by the immensity of the task of applying the *yamas* and *niyamas* to one's daily life. The initial step might seem so difficult that one would despair of ever being able to progress further. The aspirant is not, however, asked to attain perfection in the *yamas* and *niyamas* right away. Few would be capable of this. Instead, one should regard the *yamas* and *niyamas* as ideals towards which one works with sincerity. In the meantime one should attempt to observe them to the fullest extent possible. Each failure should be motivation for future success, while even a small degree of success will reduce the intensity of emotional upheavals and mental distractions.

THREE

Asanas and their Therapeutic Value

Patanjali has not described *asanas* and *pranayama* in detail. These aspects of raja yoga were developed later by the exponents of hatha yoga who realized that in order to arouse *kundalini*, the latent energy within, one has to practice and perfect *asanas* and *pranayama*, for a sickly and dissipated constitution is an obstacle when one scales the higher rungs of the yoga ladder. Hatha yoga is therefore necessary to ensure physical health and harmony—prerequisites for concentration and meditation. It is both auxiliary to raja yoga and an essential part of it.

Asana is the Sanskrit word for posture, of which there are two kinds—*asanas* for meditation and *asanas* for physical well-being. The *asanas* suitable for *pranayama*, concentration and meditation are *padmasana*—the lotus posture, *siddhasana*—the accomplished posture, *swastikasana*—the auspicious posture, *sukhasana*—the easy posture, and a few others. In all of them emphasis is placed on keeping the head, neck and trunk erect which results in a steady and comfortable posture with minimal production of carbon dioxide. This slows down the activity of the heart and lungs, and the mind is thus less disturbed by the body. This, in turn, aids concentration greatly. The other *asanas*, which aim at physical well-being, control specific muscles and nerves in the body and have specific therapeutic effects.

Photographs of some of the more important *asanas* are included in this book, but there is no detailed discussion of their practice or of the precautionary measures to be observed. A manual on hatha yoga would have to be consulted for this purpose, and personal instruction from a competent teacher is necessary in the more advanced postures. In this chapter we will consider the physiological aspects of some of these *asanas* and their value as therapeutic measures, but first we will examine those postures used for meditation and *pranayama*.

Meditative Postures

Great emphasis has been placed, in Patanjali's *Yoga Sutras* as well as in other scriptures, on cultivating a posture which is comfortable and steady, one in which the head, neck and trunk are erect and in line. If in the early stages the aspirant does not heed this injunction and assumes his own posture for concentration and meditation, he will suffer from a great handicap when trying to scale the higher rungs of the yoga ladder. Those who want to tread the path of yoga seriously and successfully should follow the order and the scientific process expounded by yogis. If the head, neck and trunk are not erect the aspirant's body begins to tremble after a few minutes, thus disturbing his mind. The trunk slowly begins to form a curve, restricting the flow of vital energy through the spinal cord, and resulting in the gland centers not being energized by the circulation of blood. Finally, an improper and restricted blood circulation upsets the respiratory system, and the aspirant will find it difficult to breathe in a natural way. So in order to avoid these problems the adepts of ancient wisdom have formulated four main postures for practicing the science of breathing, concentration and meditation. They are *padmasana*—the lotus posture, *siddhasana*—the accomplished posture, *swastikasana*—the auspicious posture and *sukhasana*—the easy posture.

Padmasana—The Lotus Posture

Sit on the floor on a rug or a blanket which has been folded a few times to provide a cushion and spread the legs forward. Now bring the head, neck and trunk into a straight line. Slowly lift the left foot with the hands and place it on the right thigh. Then place the right foot on the left thigh. Place the hands on the knees with the tip of the index finger and thumb joined to form a circle, or "finger lock." (See Figure 1). Or you may place the hands palms upward, with the tip of the index finger touching the midportion of the thumb.

If the lotus posture is uncomfortable or painful the aspirant can try one of the other postures, instead. It is used mainly in order to develop limberness in the lower extremities, but as a meditative posture it is not ordinarily used by the common practitioner. Highly accomplished yogis usually master *siddhasana*; only

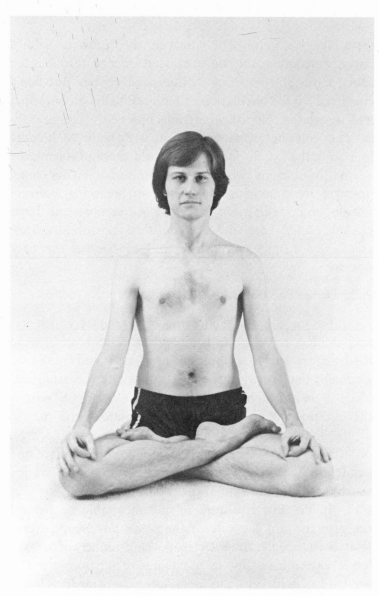

Figure 1. *Padmasana*—The Lotus Posture

rarely do a few master *padmasana*, for it is difficult to apply the root lock in this posture.

Siddhasana—The Accomplished Posture

In *siddhasana* (See Figure 2), the left heel is placed at the perineum (the region between the anus and the genitals) after the root lock has been applied (This is done by contracting the anal sphincter muscles and pulling them in.) Now the other heel is placed at the pubic bone above the organ of generation. The feet and legs are arranged so that the ankle joints are in one line, or touch each other. The toes of the right foot are placed between the left thigh and calf so that only the big toe is visible, and the toes of the left foot are pulled up between the right thigh and calf so that the big toe is visible. The hands may then be placed as in the lotus posture.

Swastikasana—The Auspicious Posture

This posture (See Figure 3) is a comfortable one and is especially recommended for women. It is similar to the accomplished posture except that the heels and ankle bones are not aligned. The left leg is bent at the knee and the left foot placed with the sole in close contact with the right thigh. The right foot is then placed on top of the left calf, with the outer edge of the foot and the toes between the thigh and calf muscles. Only the big toe should be visible. The toes of the left foot are then pulled up between the right thigh and calf so that the big toe is visible. In this way a symmetrical and stable posture is attained. The hands may be arranged as in the first two postures.

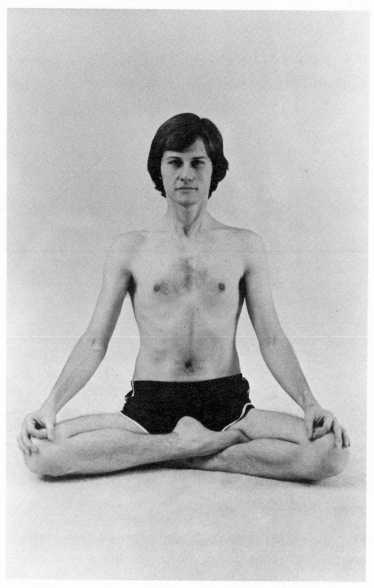

Figure 2. *Siddhasana*—The Accomplished Posture

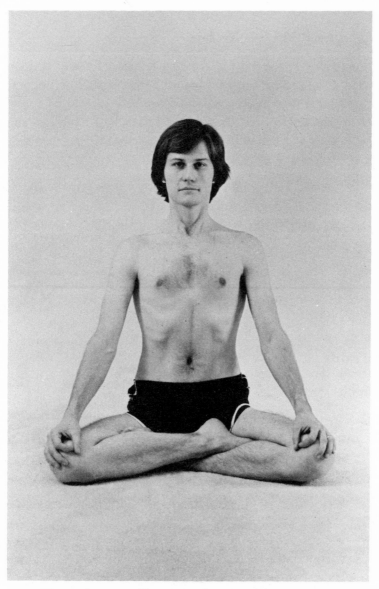

Figure 3. *Swastikasana*—The Auspicious Posture

Sukhasana—The Easy Posture

This is the simple cross-legged posture and can be used if the other three postures are painful or uncomfortable. It may also be used by beginners and older people. Here, the left foot is placed below the right knee and the right foot just below the left knee. Each knee can then rest on the opposite foot.

After mastering one of the above postures the aspirant will experience great joy in it. If there is pain in the legs after sitting in the posture for awhile, stretch the legs, massage them for a few minutes, and then resume the posture. It is quite permissible for beginners, or those who experience difficulty sitting in the time-honored postures, to sit erect in a straight-backed chair, placing the hands on the knees or thighs, and keeping the head, neck and trunk straight. Do not keep changing the posture; practice it regularly. Through continual practice of a steady posture one acquires mastery over the body and the mind.

Postures for Physical Well-being

Asanas should be performed on a carpet or folded blanket in a clean, quiet, well-ventilated room or in the open air. They may be performed in the morning or in the evening (the body is more flexible in the evening). A warm bath before the *asanas* is helpful, as it promotes circulation and reduces stiffness of the joints. The bladder and bowels must be emptied before practicing *asanas*, and at least four hours should have elapsed from the last normal-sized meal. All movements should be slow, deliberate and controlled. *Asanas* should be performed only to the extent possible; overstraining should be avoided. Patience, perseverance and regularity ensure success.

A consideration of the internal workings of the body indicates that the systems significant to physical well-being are the nervous system, the endocrine system, the circulatory system, the digestive system, the urinary system and the respiratory system. The nervous system coordinates the functions of all other systems in the body. The endocrine glands influence the nervous system and also help in maintaining the physiological balance of the different organisms. The circulatory system is responsible for transporting nourishment to all the cells of the body and for carrying away the waste products from the cells. The blood cells, which perform this function, absorb proteins, fats, sugars and salts from the digested food in the stomach and intestines and absorb oxygen from the inhaled air in the lungs. The air exhaled by the lungs carries away carbon dioxide from the blood cells while other waste products are eliminated as feces through the colon and as urine through the urinary system. Thus these different systems work together to maintain physical health, and we will now consider the beneficial influence of the *asanas* on them.

Shirshasana—The Headstand

In the headstand (See Figure 4), because it is an inverted posture, there is a rich supply of arterial blood to the brain, the cranial nerves, the pituitary gland and the pineal gland. It also provides very efficient drainage of venous blood from the legs and abdominal cavity back to the heart. We can therefore see that the brain, the nervous system, the pituitary and pineal glands, the digestive organs and the veins of the legs benefit from this *asana*. It promotes the general well-being of the individual and may be used to relieve cases of nervous debility, dyspepsia and constipation, seminal weakness and varicose veins.

1.   Sitting on your heels, bend forward, placing your forearms on the floor. The elbows should be against, or a few inches ahead of, the knees. Position the elbows slightly less (but not more) than a shoulder's width apart (the proper distance can be found by bringing the knees together and placing the elbows on the outside of each knee or by enclosing each hand around the opposite elbow). Interlock the fingers, forming a cup with the hands.

2.   Place the front of the top of the head, at about the hairline, on the well-cushioned floor. Rest the back of the head in the hands. Slowly walk the feet towards the body and bring the knees to the chest.

3.   Inhaling, raise both feet off the floor, keeping the knees to the chest in a tucked position. Become balanced and steady at this point.

4.   Keeping the knees bent, slowly raise the thighs away from the chest, bringing them up and aligning them with the trunk, letting the lower legs and feet remain limp.

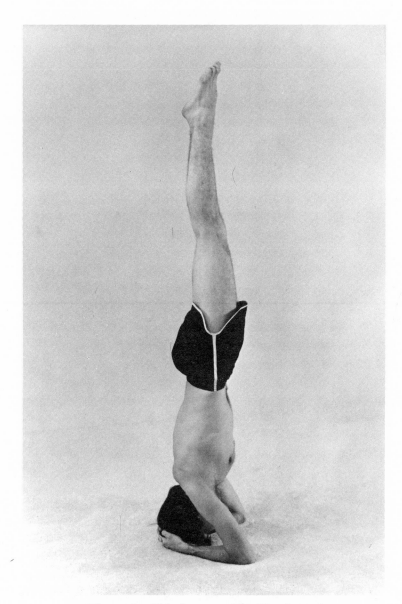

Figure 4. *Shirshasana*—The Headstand

5.   Straighten the legs, keeping the heels together, pointing the toes upwards. The weight of the body is borne on the head, forearms and elbows. Pulling in the stomach will prevent the back from arching.

6.   Become steady in the pose, concentrating on even breathing and achieving balance.

7.   Hold to your capacity, increasing up to five minutes for full benefit; then come down slowly, retracing all the steps. Relax.

Sarvangasana—The Shoulderstand

The shoulderstand (See Figure 5) stimulates the thyroid and parathyroid glands and maintains them in a healthy condition. The thyroid gland influences the functions of the whole system, so this *asana* promotes health throughout the entire body. It is therefore called *sarvangasana (sarva* in Sanskrit means "all" and *anga* means "limb"). In this *asana* the flood of blood to the brain is checked since the chin is pressed against the chest, and, as in the headstand, there is easy drainage of venous blood from the legs and abdominal cavity. This *asana* may be used to relieve nervous debility, dyspepsia and constipation, degeneration of the sex glands, hypertension, hemorrhoids, varicose veins, bronchitis, headaches, throat ailments and many other common problems. It also helps to rejuvenate the whole body and to combat the effects of old age.

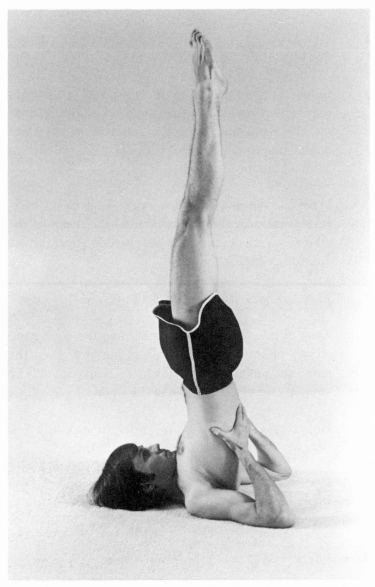

Figure 5. *Sarvangasana*—The Shoulderstand

1. Lie down on the back, arms at the sides, palms down and feet together.

2. Exhale, slowly raising both legs straight up until they are perpendicular to the floor. Lift the hips off the floor and bring the feet toward the floor behind the head. The chest should meet the chin to form a chin lock.

3. Place the palms as high up on the back as possible, fingers towards the center of the back, keeping the elbows as close together as possible, not further apart than the shoulders.

4. Exhaling, raise both legs straight up.

5. Keep the legs straight by tightening the back hamstrings of the legs and buttocks muscles. Keep the stomach pulled in. The whole body should be straight and perpendicular to the floor.

6. Hold to your capacity. In order to gain the full benefits of the posture, hold five minutes.

7. Lower the arms to the floor, palms down. Then slowly lower the back to the floor, one vertebra at a time.

8. Inhale, and lower the legs to the floor.

9. Relax and breathe deeply, lying flat on the back.

Matsyasana—The Fish Posture

This *asana* (See Figure 6) is complementary to the shoulderstand and always follows it. Only then does one achieve the full benefit of the shoulderstand. *Matsyasana* also stimulates the thyroid and parathyroid glands; it eliminates stiffness in the neck and back, and increases blood circulation to the face and neck. Since the chest is expanded the breathing becomes fuller. The pelvic joints also become more flexible. This *asana* is used to relieve common colds and inflamed tonsils as well as inflamed and bleeding hemorrhoids.

1. Assume the lotus posture (see page 33).

2. Lie on the back; do not allow the knees to be raised from the floor.

3. Exhale completely; then, inhaling, raise up on the elbows, lifting the chest and head from the floor. Allow the head to fall backward, and rest the top of the head on the floor. Keeping the upper back arched and the chest expanded, allow the weight of the trunk to rest on the top of the head, stretching the neck. The hands may take hold of the toes. Breathe deeply.

4. Again support the body with the elbows, and with an exhalation, loosen the pressure on the head and neck, lowering completely to the floor. Relax.

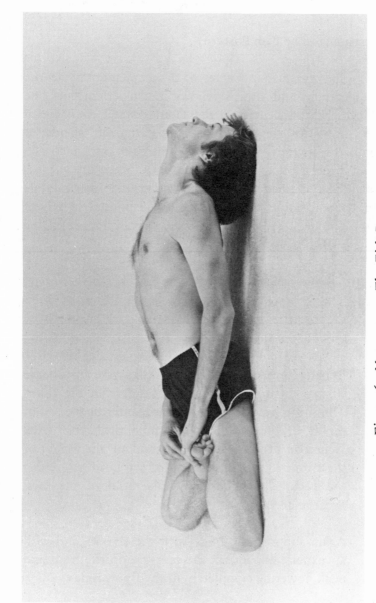

Figure 6. *Matsyasana*—The Fish Posture

Halasana—The Plough Posture

This posture (See Figure 7) benefits the spine and spinal nerves greatly—and a youthful spine connotes a youthful body. It also stimulates the thyroid and parathyroid glands, (though to a lesser extent than the shoulderstand), and contracts the abdominal muscles, which lead to a healthy digestive system. This *asana* may be used to correct deviations of the spine, combat constipation, help arthritis of the back, rejuvenate the digestive organs, sex glands and kidneys, alleviate headaches and eliminate fatigue.

1. Lie on the back, feet together and palms on the floor.

2. Slowly raise the legs until they are perpendicular to the floor. Lift the trunk and, keeping the legs straight and close together, lower the toes to the floor as close to the head as possible. All movements should be performed slowly and gracefully.

3. After this stage has been maintained for a few seconds, the toes should be pushed further beyond the head, feeling pressure, first at the lower dorsal region, then at the upper dorsal region and last in the cervical region when the pose is fully extended. This position presses the chin tightly to form a perfect chin lock.

4. Place the arms over the head, fingers pointing

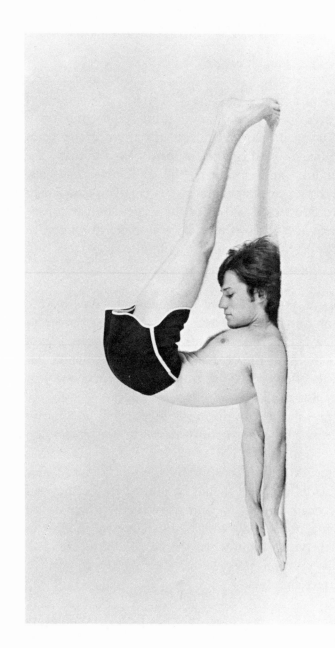

Figure 7. *Halasana*—The Plough Posture

towards the toes, and breathe deeply.

5.   Return the toes again to the original position near the head. Maintain the pose twenty to thirty seconds in this position. Then retrace all the steps in coming out of the pose. Relax.

Bhujangasana—The Cobra Posture
Shalabhasana—The Locust Posture
Dhanurasana—The Bow Posture

These three postures (See Figures 8, 9, 10) have been grouped together, as they are similar in that they give the spine a backward bend and stretch the abdominal muscles. In the cobra posture, and to a lesser extent in the bow posture, the deep muscles of the back are exercised. Blood circulation to the back muscles, the spine and spinal nerves, and the abdominal organs is greatly promoted. The chest is also expanded in these *asanas* so that breathing becomes fuller. The locust posture requires retention of the breath, and the resulting high pressure in the lungs helps in maintaining their elasticity. These *asanas* also prevent functional disturbances of the stomach, liver, kidneys and intestines and may be used to combat constipation, lumbago, gastric trouble, flatulence and backaches. The locust and bow postures may also be used to correct deviations of the spine and slipped discs.

Bhujangasana—The Cobra Posture

1.   Lie on your stomach, forehead on the floor.

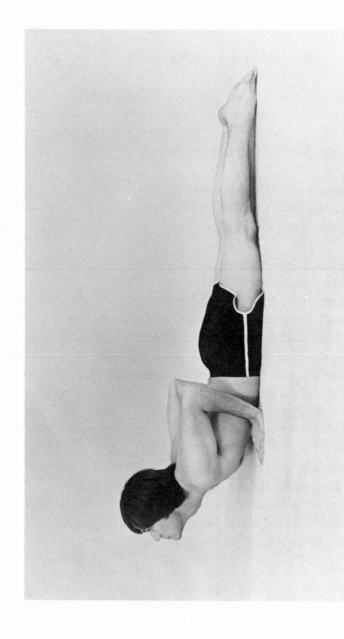

Figure 8. *Bhujangasana*—The Cobra

2. Place your palms alongside the breasts, keeping the elbows close to the body. The toes point away from the body, with the heels together.

3. With an inhalation, slowly raise the head, then the neck and chest, one vertebra at a time, using only the muscles of the back. Keep the navel on the floor (the abdominal muscles will press into the floor). The legs should be relaxed, heels together. The arms should not bear any weight; only the lower back muscles should be used to raise and hold the pose.

4. Hold to your capacity.

5. With an exhalation, slowly lower the chest to the floor, one vertebra at a time.

6. Relax with deep, even breathing.

Shalabhasana—The Locust Posture

1. Lie on your stomach, resting your chin on the floor. The toes are pointing away from the body, heels together. Arms are at the sides, palms up.

2. Make a fist and position the hands alongside, or just underneath, the thighs.

3. Inhale, and slowly raise both legs together off the floor, keeping them straight.   Then, in the same

motion, tense the arms, pressing the forearms into the floor, thus raising the navel off the floor and the legs still higher.

4.   Hold as long as the breath can be comfortably retained.

5.   Exhale, and slowly lower the legs to the floor.

6.   Relax with even breathing.

Dhanurasana—The Bow Posture

1.   Lie on the stomach; rest the chin on the floor and the arms at the sides.

2.   Bend the legs at the knees and bring the heels close to the buttocks.

3.   Reach back and grasp the right ankle with the right hand and the left ankle with the left hand.

4.   Inhaling and retaining the breath, raise the chin, head and chest up, simultaneously raising the thighs and hips. Keeping the knees together, try to straighten the legs without releasing the hands. The whole body stretches up, resting on the abdomen.

5.   Hold for as long as the breath can be comfortably retained.

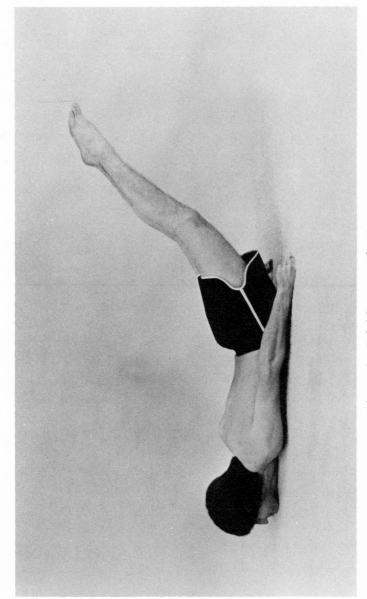

Figure 9. *Salabhasana*—The Locust

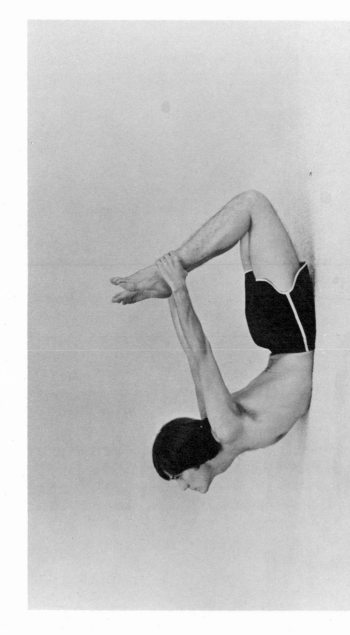

Figure 10. *Dhanurasana*—The Bow Posture

6.   Exhaling, slowly lower the body to the floor and release the ankles. Relax.

Ardha-Matsyendrasana—The Spinal Twist

This posture (See Figure 11) is useful as a spinal exercise because it gives a sideways twist to the spine in both directions. It therefore has a beneficial effect on the whole nervous system. In addition, blood circulation to the abdominal organs is improved and the abdominal muscles are strengthened. This *asana* may be used to relieve lumbago, displaced shoulder joints, sprains in the neck and shoulder muscles, a congested liver, a congested spleen and inactive kidneys.

1.   Sit on the floor with the legs outstretched in front of you. Bend the right leg at the knee and place the heel against the perineum.

2.   Bending the left leg, raise the knee up and cross the left foot over the right thigh, placing it firmly on the floor, the ankle against the knee.

3.   Inhale and stretch the ribs up. Turn the trunk to the left. Raise the right arm over the left knee and bring the chest against the left thigh. The back of the shoulder and upper arm will press against the left knee and thigh. Place the left arm on the floor behind the left hip for balance.

4.   Inhaling and twisting still more, grasp the instep

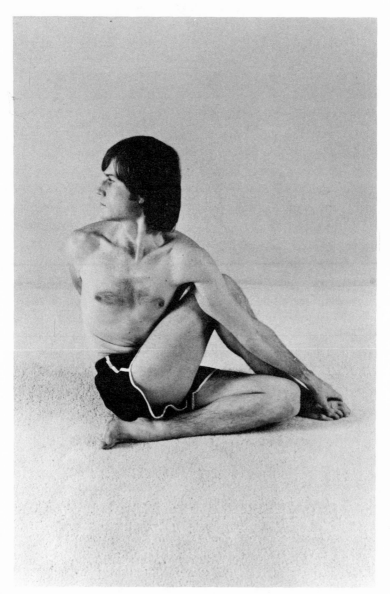

Figure 11. *Ardha-Matsyendrasana*—The Spinal Twist

of the left foot with the right hand and push the left knee further to the right. Turn the head, bringing the chin almost in line with the left shoulder. Reach across the back with the left arm and hold the right thigh just below the hip joint.

5. Breathe deeply; holding the posture to your capacity; then repeat the process on the opposite side in order to balance the twist to the spine.

Mayurasana—The Peacock Posture

This *asana* (See Figure 12) strengthens the forearms, wrists and elbows and gives a liberal blood supply to the digestive organs. It also increases intra-abdominal pressure, thus benefiting digestive organs and stimulating the nerves of the abdominal cavity. *Mayurasana* also helps to eliminate toxins in the body and combats ailments of the stomach, spleen and pancreas.

1. Sit on the heels and spread the knees apart. Place the palms on the floor between the legs, elbows together, thumbs out, fingers extended and pointing back. Bring the forearms together from the wrists to the elbows, providing a fulcrum on which to support the body. Press the elbows against the abdomen at the navel.

2. Bend forward, placing the forehead on the floor. Straighten the legs out behind, bringing the weight of the body onto the arms and the elbows.

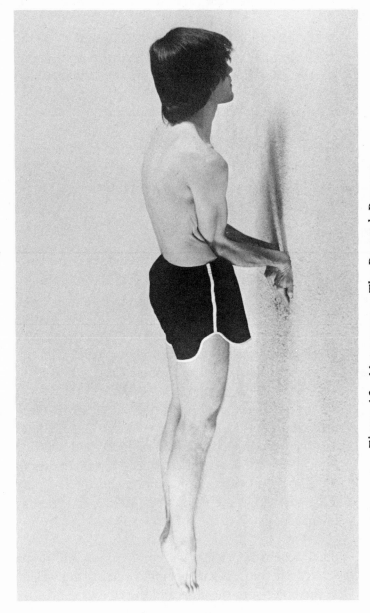

Figure 12. *Mayurasana*—The Peacock Posture

3.   Inhale, and gently come slightly forward onto the elbows, tightening the abdominal muscles and at the same time arching the lower back and raising the legs from the floor. The forearms are at a right angle to the floor and inclined slightly to the front. The head is raised and the chin thrown out to counter-balance the weight of the legs. In this position the body is held like a bar resting on a fulcrum, perfectly straight and parallel to the floor.

4.   Hold to your capacity with retention of breath.

5.   Exhaling, lower the forehead to the floor. Bring the legs back underneath you and sit on your heels. Relax with even breathing.

Paschimottanasana—The Posterior Stretch

This posture (See Figure 13) stretches the muscles of the back and the hamstring muscles at the back of the knees. The front abdominal muscles are contracted, the pelvic and lumbrosacral nerves are benefited, the spine is rendered supple and the heart is massaged. This *asana* may be used to relieve malfunctioning of the stomach, liver, kidneys and intestines, disorders of the sex glands, and to reduce the waist and hips.

1.   Sit on the floor with the legs outstretched in front of you.

2.   Inhaling, stretch the arms over the head, pulling the

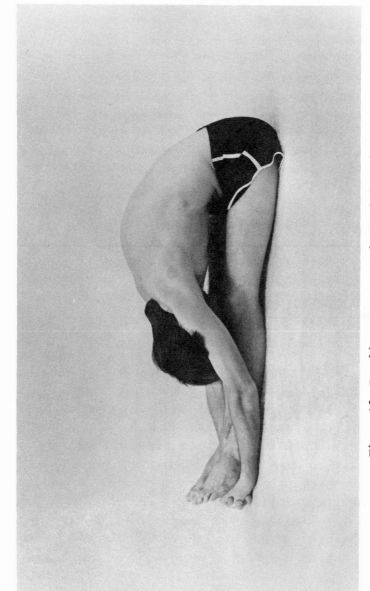

Figure 13. *Paschimottanasana*—The Back Stretch

spine straight up. The palms should face forward.

3.   Exhaling, bend forward at the hip joints (not the waist).

4.   Keeping the spine straight, reach and grasp the toes, ankles or calves, according to your capacity. Keep the legs straight and the back part of the knees flat on the floor. Try to stretch down until the chest and stomach lie on the thighs and the forehead, nose or chin rests on the knees.

5.   Catch hold of the toes, with the arms slightly bent and the elbows touching the floor alongside the legs, but do not use your arms to pull you forward. Use the weight of the trunk to press the legs against the floor.

6.   Hold to your capacity with even breathing, relaxing into the posture.

7.   With an inhalation, raise back up to the starting position. Then relax completely.

Yoga Mudra—The Symbol of Yoga

This *asana* (See Figure 14) has many of the benefits of the posterior stretch. It also helps to reposition displaced abdominal organs because of the pressure of the heels against the cecum and pelvic loop. It expands the chest and increases the range of shoulder movements.

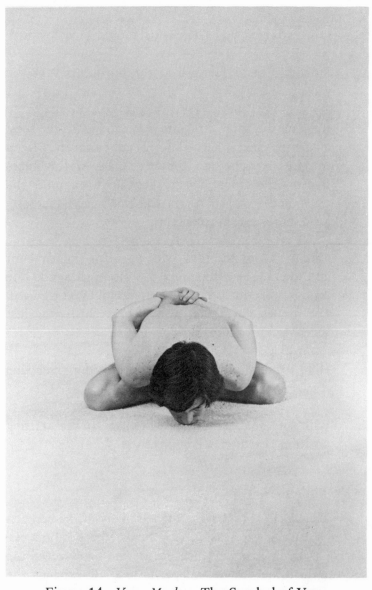

Figure 14. *Yoga Mudra*—The Symbol of Yoga

Peristaltic activity is intensified. This *asana* is helpful for constipation and seminal weakness.

1. Assume the lotus posture. If this cannot be done, then either the half lotus or easy posture is acceptable. Reach behind the back with both hands, interlacing the fingers. Keep the spine erect.

2. Exhaling, bend forward from the hip joints and keep the back straight. Rest the forehead on the floor in front of the legs. Do not allow the buttocks to lift off the floor. Let the breath become deep and even, holding the pose to your capacity.

3. With an inhalation, and keeping the trunk straight, return to a sitting position. Release the hands and stretch the legs. Relax.

Chakrasana—The Wheel Posture

Through this *asana* (See Figure 15) the body becomes very supple and alert. The arms and wrists are strengthened and the muscles of the legs, hips, shoulders and ligaments of the spine are stretched.

1. Lie on the back, feet slightly apart. Bend the knees and rest the spine flat on the floor. Place the hands on the floor next to the head, palms down, thumb side towards the head with the fingers pointing towards the toes.

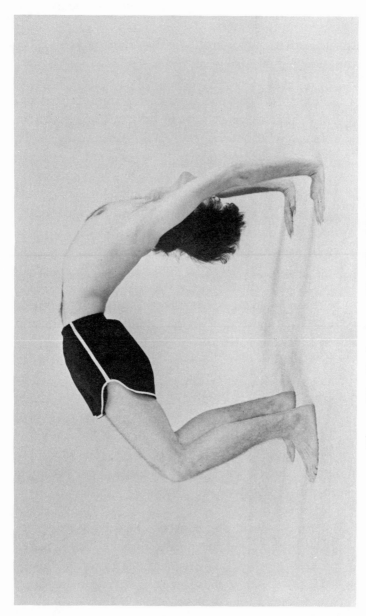

Figure 15. *Chakrasana*—The Wheel Posture

2. Inhaling, lift the body to rest on the top of the head, then straighten the arms and arch the back. Walk the feet towards the head but do not come up onto the toes. Push the abdomen upwards and gaze at the floor between the hands. The closer the feet are to the hands, the greater the curve of the back.

3. Breathe deeply, holding the pose to your capacity. Then, exhaling, slowly lower the body to the floor. Relax.

Vrischikasana—The Scorpion Posture

In this posture (See Figure 16) the abdominal muscles are stretched, the lungs expanded and the spine maintained in a healthy condition.

1. Sitting on the heels, bend forward, raising up onto the knees, and place the forearms on the floor, elbows six to eight inches in front of the knees, palms down and fingers relaxed. The forearms should be the width of the head apart at the wrists and parallel to each other, or slightly further apart at the elbows. Reposition the feet onto the toes and the balls of the feet. Raise the head up, fixing the gaze on the floor well ahead of the finger tips.

2. Lift both knees from the floor, raising the buttocks up. Raise one leg up as high as possible, then gently spring up off the floor with a slight push from the

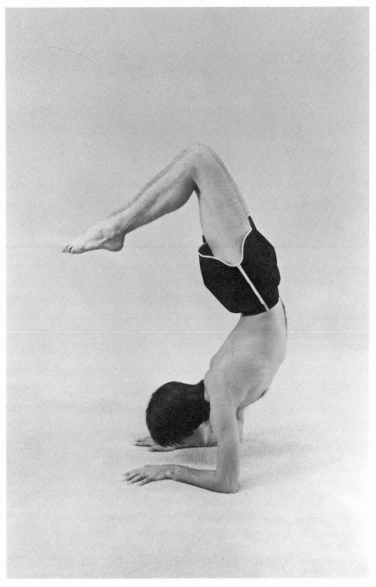

Figure 16. *Vrischikasana*—The Scorpion Posture

other leg. Bring both legs up, arching the back, and bring the legs together, coming to a point of balance. Bend the knees so that the toes reach toward the back of the head.

3. Hold to your capacity; breathe evenly.

4. Slowly lower the body, bending at the waist, bringing one foot to the floor first and then the other. Lower to the knees, sitting on the heels, and rest the forehead on the floor. Relax completely with even breathing.

Ustrasana—The Camel Posture

The spine is stretched and toned in this posture (See Figure 17) which is helpful for drooping shoulders and hunched backs.

1. Sit on the heels with the knees together and the back straight. Reach back and place the palms of the hands on the soles of the feet.

2. Inhaling, and without losing the contact between the hands and feet, lift the buttocks off the heels and lift the hips as far up and forward as possible. Drop the head back and gaze at the point between the eyebrows, or close the eyes. If possible, move the hands from the feet and grasp the ankles.

3. There is a tendency to hold the breath (as in all

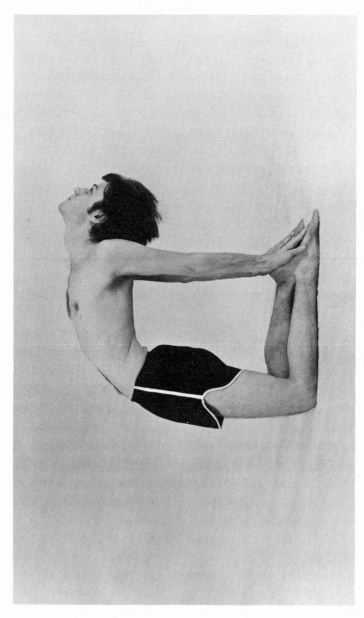

Figure 17. *Ustrasana*—The Camel Posture

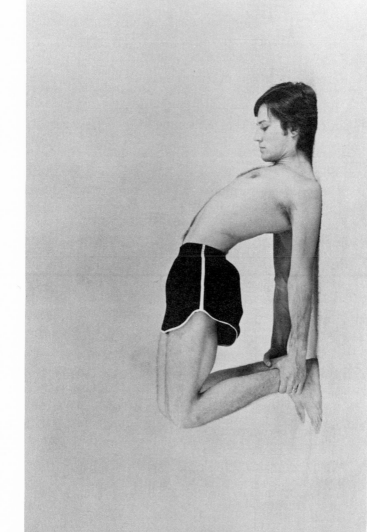

Figure 18. *Setu-bandhasana*—The Bridge Posture

backward bending postures), so an effort must be made to be sure that you are breathing deeply.

4.   Return to a sitting position. Relax.

Setu-bandhasana—The Bridge Posture

This *asana* (See Figure 18) strengthens the neck as well as the extensor muscles of the back and spine. In addition, the pineal, pituitary, thyroid and adrenal glands are benefited by the increased supply of blood to them.

1.   Lie on the back. Bring the feet to the buttocks, with the knees up, and grasp the ankles, keeping the knees and ankles together and feet flat on the floor.

2.   Inhaling, lift the hips from the floor and arch the back up, stretching the front of the thighs and contracting the buttocks. The shoulders and head should remain on the floor. Breathe deeply and evenly while in the posture.

3.   Hold to your capacity.

4.   Exhale, and lower the hips to the floor. Release the ankles, stretch the legs out straight and relax in the corpse posture.

Shavasana—The Corpse Posture

This *asana* (See Figure 19) relaxes the body. It is

used in between the different *asanas* and after all of them have been performed. In this posture all muscle tension is reduced, venous circulation is improved, the whole nervous system toned and fatigue relieved. In addition, the heart is rested and the distribution of blood is uniform. The breathing becomes slow, deep and rhythmic. This *asana* is used to cure degeneration of the nerves as well as high blood pressure.

1. Lie on the back. Spread the feet apart slightly. Place the arms out at your sides, palms up. Do not allow one limb to touch another. Close your eyes.

2. Relax all the muscles of the body. Let the body and mind be perfectly still. Breathe from the diaphragm —slowly and deeply. Be both mentally alert and relaxed.

The essential difference between *asanas* and other systems of physical culture should now be evident. While other systems aim at merely developing a muscular body, hatha yoga aims at promoting the health of the internal organs as well. Thus, complete physical harmony is achieved, and this is an essential prerequisite to achieving one-pointedness of mind. But the main reason hatha yoga is important is that it is preparatory training for the higher rungs of the yoga ladder.

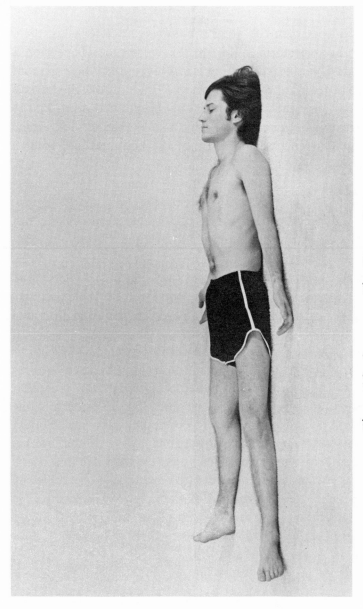

Figure 19. *Savasana*—The Corpse Posture

Internal Cleansing

In addition to the postures, there are a number of *kriyas*, or cleansing exercises, involved in hatha yoga. *Kriya* means "preliminary" or "preparatory," and these techniques free the body, leaving one feeling refreshed and purified of excess mucus and other wastes. Thus they prepare the student for the practice of meditation. Although the idea of cleaning the interior of the body may not be appealing at first, once the student experiences the invigoration and feeling of lightness that it brings, and sees the freedom from colds and chronic ailments that can result, he begins to take pleasure in them. To the practitioner who has refined his sensitivity to internal processes, the practices of internal cleansing become as important as bathing is to most people.

A few of the most basic *kriyas* will be described. They should be practiced in the morning, shortly after arising, before doing the hatha yoga *asanas* and, of course, before eating.

Jala Neti—Nasal Wash

This is a technique for removing excess mucus from the nasal and sinus passages. It clears obstructions so that the breath can flow freely through the nostrils, and this helps prevent colds and relieves the symptoms of hayfever and other allergies. Variations of this practice are now recommended by some physicians.

1.   Place half a cup of tepid water into a small vessel

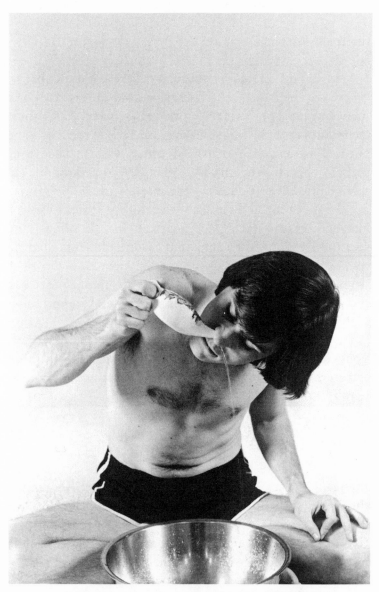

Figure 20. *Jala Neti*—The Nasal Wash

which has a long spout. Add a pinch of salt to the water—the proper amount of salt should produce a solution that tastes like tears. This degree of saltiness has a soothing effect on the linings of the nose and throat and will prevent the water from causing a burning sensation in the nasal passages.

2.   Stand over a sink and tilt the head to the right. Place the spout against the left nostril and slowly pour the water into the nostril. If the head is tilted at the proper angle the water will run out of the opposite nostril. (See Figure 20).

3.   Repeat the same procedure, pouring the water into the right nostril.

4.   Remove excess water from the nasal passages.

Sutra Neti—String Cleansing

Here, a length of good quality, sterilized cotton cord is used to clean the nasal passages. In addition to removing excess mucus and keeping the nostrils free of obstruction, this practice facilitates the proper flow of air and thereby makes the practice of breathing exercises easier. It decreases the likelihood of developing ailments of the upper respiratory passages as well, and improves such conditions as sinusitis and weak vision.

1.   A length of good quality sterilized cotton cord is unravelled on one end, while the other end is

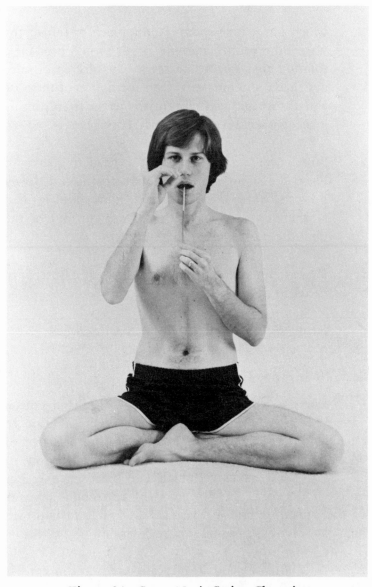

Figure 21. *Sutra Neti*—String Cleansing

dipped in beeswax. As this end stiffens it should be made blunt by shaping.

2. Insert the blunt end gently, like a probe, into the nostril several inches so that it enters the passage coming down toward the throat. (During the first few attempts, tearing and sneezing may be induced; this subsides with practice, however.)

3. When the end of the string is felt at the base of the tongue, reach inside the mouth with the thumb and index finger, grasping the blunt end and pulling it out through the mouth. The other end remains in the nostril. (See Figure 21).

4. Move the threads back and forth slowly, gently opening and cleaning the nasal passages.

5. Remove the string and repeat the process in the other nostril.

Gajakarani—Upper Wash

The upper wash is an exercise that cleans the stomach and bronchial passages. It is performed by swallowing a large quantity of water, then throwing it out. The upward pressure not only empties the stomach, it also forces accumulated mucus from the respiratory passages. It has been proven effective in some respiratory diseases as well as in some gastric disorders.

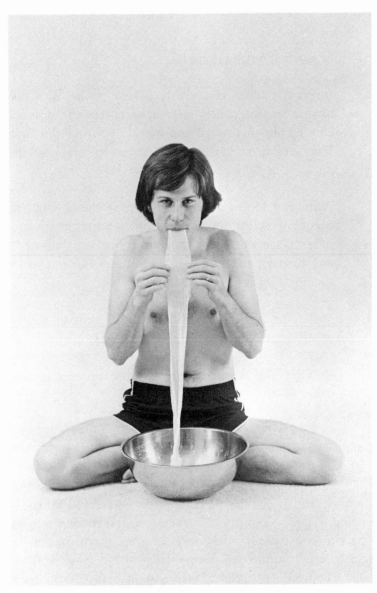

Figure 22. *Dhauti*—Cleansing with Cloth

1. The stomach should be empty (unless the *kriya* is performed to clear the digestive tract of undesirable food).

2. Prepare four to six quarts of lukewarm water and add enough salt to make it taste somewhat stronger than tears.

3. While in a squatting position, drink the water as rapidly as possible, with no pause or interruption.

4. By the time the amount has been taken, regurgitation will often occur spontaneously. If not, stand up, lean forward over a basin, insert the fingers in the throat and gently stimulate the back of the tongue, simultaneously pushing and massaging the upper abdomen with the other hand. Be careful not to scratch or injure the throat with the fingernails.

5. All the water should be thrown out. When first performing the exercise it is helpful to measure the amount of water taken in as well as that thrown up.

6. Afterwards, take only juices for several hours. A heavy meal should not be taken for some time.

Dhauti—Cleansing with Cloth

This practice removes excess mucus from the esophagus and stomach where it tends to accumulate as a result of the constant swallowing of drainage from sinuses, nasal passages and bronchi.

1.   Use a three-inch wide strip of very fine white cotton cloth, twenty-two to twenty-three feet in length for this practice (the beginner may use a shorter cloth).

2.   Sterilize the cloth by boiling it in water.

3.   Grasp one end of the cloth, spreading it out and placing it as far back on the tongue as possible.

4.   Begin swallowing the cloth as you continue to spread it and feed it into the mouth (See Figure 22). If the cloth does not go down, swallowing a few sips of water will often help to get it started.

5.   Continue swallowing until you are holding only six inches of the cloth outside the mouth.

6.   Pull the cloth out rapidly, allowing the natural gag reflex to help throw it (and the accompanying mucus) out.

FOUR

Pranayama

When a student starts practicing postures accurately he becomes more aware of variations in the flow of his breath, and then the teacher can begin to give him various tehcniques of breathing exercises, or *pranayama*. The meaning of the word *pranayama* may be explained in two ways: *Prana* is energy, or the life force, and *yama* means the control of that energy. Or the word *pranayama* may be divided into *prana* and *ayama*. In this case *ayama* means expansion, or rising, so *pranayama* may be understood as the practice whereby the flow of *prana* is made more extensive and expansive as well as being brought under control.

The word *prana* is composed of two words, *pra* and *na*. *Pra* means "first unit" and *na* means "energy." This first unit of energy is in its subtlest aspect in man; the universe is its expansion. Thus, there is no qualitative difference between man and the universe. The underlying principle in both is *prana* and *prana* is the sum total of all energy that is manifest in man and in the universe. In the beginning there was *akasha*, or space, and through *prana* the universe was manifest. All that is present in the world of sense perception is only an expression and manifestation of this vital energy. It is *prana* that feeds and sustains the mind and produces thoughts. It is therefore related to the mind, through mind to the will, through will to the individual *atman* and thus to the cosmic soul, *Brahman.* All sensations, all thinking, feeling and knowing are possible only because of *prana.*

The science of breath is an important part of the science of *pranayama*, but the world has not yet recognized this important aspect of life. Yogis alone know the secret of this science, for the subject is vast and recondite. Many talk of physical health. Others talk of the soul, the universe and God. But the real mystery of *prana* remains veiled even though it is *prana* which sustains the body, and without its help body and mind could not exist.

Modern science has done much research on diet, calories, vitamins and minerals. The mind and its functions are also being studied. The breath links the body and the mind, and very little research has been done on the science of breath. There are many books on philosophy and religion, but few books deal with *pranayama* because it must be known experientially and only one who has mastered its practices can explain it thoroughly.

Prana sustains life. It enters the body through the food we eat and the air we breathe. The vital part of food is *prana*, without which none can live, even for a few minutes, but food contains a grosser quality of *prana* than does the breath, which carries it in a more subtle form. In other words, the vital energy, or *prana*, contained in the food we eat is important, but even more indispensable is the vital energy contained in the air we breathe. There is no medicine known to man which can substitute for this vital energy which we absorb through our food and breath. It is important to remember, though, that *prana* is not the air we breathe or the food we eat; they are merely vehicles. So just as man takes in food, vitamins, protein and calories, so he should learn and practice the most important and vital exercise of filling his lungs completely at least twice a day.

Regulating the lungs is the most vital process in cleansing the human system. When our lungs go into action an exchange takes place between the vital *prana* that is being consumed and that *prana* which has already been consumed. Overeating, or eating overcooked food disrupts this exchange, and both the lungs and the entire respiratory system become irregular. Even the pores suffer. When one regulates the motion of the lungs by certain breathing exercises, however, the pores function properly and the tissues and cells become healthy.

The lungs are situated on each side of the chest, with the heart, the great blood vessels and the esophagus separating them, and the air passages leading to them. At the base of the lungs we find the diaphragm, the muscular wall dividing the chest cavity from the abdomen, and it is the action of the diaphragm which draws air into the lungs. The diaphragm contracts, causing the lungs to expand, and creates a partial vacuum into which the air rushes. When the diaphragm relaxes the lungs contract and the air is expelled. So control of the diaphragm is the first step in the practice of breathing exercises. The simple practice of deep breathing with diaphragmatic movement is the foundation for the science of breath.

The air we inhale helps all the systems in our body to conduct their respective functions, and in controlling the motion of our lungs we are regulating the exchange in the storehouse of vital energies. Furthermore, by controlling the motion of the lungs, highly accomplished yogis can control the autonomic nervous system and its set of muscles. The functioning of *prana* is the basic principle underlying the systolic and diastolic actions of the heart, the exhalation and inhalation of the lungs, the digestion of food, the excretion of urine and fecal matter, and the manufacture of gastric juice, bile, intestinal juice and saliva.

By controlling the motion of the lungs one can also control the functioning of the pores, which is necessary in cleansing the whole body. The yoga manual, called *Tarangini*, explains such a method of cleansing called the *prana* bath. In order to do this, one pushes in the diaphragm, expelling the carbon dioxide and carbonic acid, without inhaling, for some time. This is done repeatedly, according to the capacity of the lungs, but it should be practiced only under the guidance of a competent and accomplished teacher. The student first needs to be skilled in some preliminary steps of *pranayama*. When practiced by advanced students the *prana* bath is one of the most effective cleansing techniques known and is highly regarded by the yogis dwelling in the Himalayan mountains.

Through knowledge of the breathing system one can control all of the motions of the body and mind. Through the practice of *pranayama* one can shape one's character and even change the course of one's life, for the knowledge of breath behavior is a very subtle and complete knowledge of the functioning of the mind and body. A number of diseases ordinarily thought to be incurable can be helped through the practices of *pranayama*, for *prana* links the physical and mental life. When this link is broken, death takes place.

It was said by the ancient sages, "One who knows the science of breathing knows everything, and he who knows *prana* knows the Vedas." For this very reason, "breath is *Brahman*." Whatever moves or works or has life is but an expression or manifestation of *prana*. It is *prana* that moves the mind, and through the mind it moves the will. *Prana* is related, through the will, to the individual soul and, in turn, to the supreme being, the cosmic soul.

In order to understand the science of *pranayama* it is necessary to consider the nature and functions of the nervous system which coordinates the functions of all the other systems in the body. It may be subdivided into the central nervous system and the autonomic nervous system. The central nervous system, also called the cerebrospinal system, consists of the brain, twelve pairs of cranial nerves, the spinal cord and thirty-one pairs of spinal nerves. The spinal cord, situated in the hollow of the spinal column, is a prolongation of the brain; the cranial nerves from the brain and the spinal nerves from the spinal cord spread throughout the body, forming a network of nerve fibers which are either efferent or afferent. Efferent fibers carry nerve impulses from the brain and spinal cord outward to the nerve endings, while afferent fibers carry nerve impulses from nerve endings inward to the brain and spinal cord.

The autonomic nervous system regulates processes in our body which are not normally under our voluntary control—processes such as the secretions of the digestive organs, the beating of the heart and the movement of the lungs. The autonomic system is further subdivided into the sympathetic and parasympathetic nervous systems. As the names suggest, these two systems work in opposition to each other and complement one another. In this way they maintain balance. For example, the parasympathetic system operates to slow down the action of the heart, while the sympathetic system accelerates the action of the heart. The regulation of heart beat results from these two opposing actions.

The sympathetic nervous system consists mainly of two rows of ganglia, or nerve cell clusters connected by cords made up of nerve fibers, arranged vertically on either side of the spinal column. Branches from these gangliated cords spread out to different glands and viscera in the thorax and abdomen and form plexuses.

The main part of the parasympathetic system is the vagus nerve which supplies and controls all the important vital organs through the different plexuses of the sympathetic system. The vagus, or "wandering" nerve, is the tenth cranial nerve and is connected with the hindbrain. It travels downward, along the spinal cord, through the neck, chest and abdomen, sending out branches to the various plexuses of the sympathetic system. Though it ends at the solar plexus it is connected with the lower plexuses through filaments. The vagus is composed of both efferent and afferent fibers, the efferent being inhibitory in action and the afferent being acceleratory. The efferent fibers influence the larynx, pharynx, lungs and heart and originate at the base of the skull from the medulla oblongata. The afferent fibers influence the stomach, intestines and blood vessels of the abdominal viscera and originate in the solar plexus. Stimulation of the vagus nerve simultaneously sets into action the inhibitory action of the efferent fibers and the acceleratory action of the afferent fibers.

The science of *pranayama* is intimately connected with the functions of the autonomic nervous system, and its techniques are aimed at bringing the functions of the autonomic system, normally considered involuntary, under conscious control. This can be achieved by regulating the breath and, through the breath, controlling the motion of the lungs, the most vital step in controlling the heart rhythm and the vagus nerve. These, in turn, bring the autonomic nervous system under perfect control, and this opens the way for experiencing the higher and subtler levels of mind. Highly accomplished yogis can also control the central nervous system so that diseases such as muscular dystrophy and Parkinson's disease can be prevented. In other words, by regulating the breath the various vehicles responsible for conducting their respective duties in our body are regulated, good health is provided and the student is led to subtler levels of awareness.

The ancient manuals of yoga science describe in detail the internal structure of the human body and its functions, and even though ancient yogis did not dissect the human body, their description of the nervous system is consistent with that of modern physiology. There is, however, one major difference between the ancient descriptions and modern ones. The description of the human body given by the ancient yogis does not refer directly to the physical details of the nervous system, but to subtler counterparts of these physical details. Their descriptions speak of *nadis*, or energy channels, and *pranas*, or vital energies, and are consistent with details of nerves and nerve impulses, respectively. In other words, physical nerves and impulses are gross manifestations of the subtler *nadis* and *pranas* that were known to the ancient yogis. Similarly, physical plexuses and gland centers are gross manifestations of the *chakras*, or spiritual centers, described by yogis.

Let us consider briefly the description given in ancient yogic manuals. There are several thousand *nadis*, of which the three main ones are *ida, pingala* and *sushumna. Sushumna* is centrally located and passes through the *merudanda* (which corresponds to the physical spinal column). It originates at the *muladhara chakra* (which corresponds to the pelvic plexus of the sympathetic system). As it passes through the *merudanda* it pierces the *swadisthana chakra* (corresponding to the hypogastric plexus), the *manipura chakra* (corresponding to the solar plexus), the *anahata chakra* (corresponding to the cardiac plexus), and the *vishuddha chakra* (corresponding to the pharynegeal plexus). The *sushumna* then pierces the *talu* (corresponding to the base of the skull), and then divides into an anterior portion and a posterior portion. The anterior portion goes toward the *ajna chakra* (corresponding to the nasociliary plexus) and joints the *brahma-randhra*, or cavity of *Brahma*, (which corresponds to the ventricular cavity in the physical body). The posterior portion of the *sushumna* passes from behind the skull and joins the *brahma-randhra*. It is this posterior portion that is developed through *pranayama*, and the realized yogi liberates his soul through the *brahma-randhra*.

The *ida* and *pingala* are on the left and right side, respectively, of the *merudanda*. They also originate in the *muladhara chakra*, and the two *nadis* cross each other before they end at the nostrils; the *ida* ends in the left nostril and the *pingala* in the right nostril.

There are detailed descriptions in yogic manuals of the *chakras*, which are centers of *pranic* energy, and which are represented as lotuses. Each *chakra* has a certain number of petals, a certain color, a presiding deity, and so on, associated with it. In the lowest center, the *muladhara chakra*, is the sleeping serpent-like fire, *kundalini* which represents all the latent potential in man. It is the aim of yoga to arouse the sleeping *kundalini* and lead it upwards through the *sushumna*, piercing the different *chakras*, to the *sahasrara chakra*, the thousand-petaled lotus at the top of the head. This represents the union of the cosmic potency, or Shakti with cosmic consciousness, or *Shiva*. Through this final union the yogi achieves realization and liberation from all bondage. He thus merges his soul, or *atman*, with the cosmic soul, *Brahman*.

Pranayama practices are the means to this awakening. They aim at devitalizing the *ida* and *pingala* and allowing the *prana*, or vital energy, to flow through the *sushumna*. The yogi then experiences unique joy and is freed from the bondage of time.

In the human body the cosmic force, *prana* was recognized by the ancients and subdivided on the basis of the ten functions it performs, and it is through the manifestation of these *pranas*, or vital energies, in the body that all bodily functions are possible and can be coordinated. These are the vehicles that transport and supply the different organs of the body with the cosmic energy. Of the ten *pranas*, there are five main *pranas: udana, prana, samana, apana, vyana.*

Udana rules the region of the body above the larynx; it governs the use of our senses. *Prana* rules the region between the larynx and the base of the heart and governs the verbal mechanism and vocal apparatus, the respiratory system and the muscles engaged in it. *Samana* rules in the regions between the heart and the navel and governs all the metabolic activity involved in digestion. *Apana* has its abode below the navel and governs the functions of the kidneys, the colon, the rectum, the bladder and the genitals. *Vyana* pervades the whole body and governs the relaxation and contraction of all muscles, voluntary and involuntary, as well as the movement of the joints and the structure around them.

In the process of *pranayama* cosmic energy, as *prana*, enters the body through the vehicle of oxygen and then, during inhalation, as *vyana*, reaches all the cells of the body and carries away waste products from them. During exhalation the force of *apana* expels the waste products through the vehicle of carbon dioxide. The cessation of the movements of inhalation and exhalation and their union is called *pranayama*—the process by which the secret of *prana* and its control is understood. On attaining this union the yogi subjugates his mind and body and grasps the very core of cosmic life.

Breath is an external manifestation of the force of *prana*. Breath is the fly-wheel that regulates the entire machine of the body. Just as the control of the fly-wheel of an engine controls all other mechanisms in it, so the control of the external breath leads to control of the gross and subtle, physical and mental aspects of our life machine.

If *prana* ceased to exist, thoughts would never arise, for the relationship between *prana* and the mind is that of the supporter and the supported. It is the relationship between a flower and its fragrance. A comprehensive knowledge of *pranayama* is, therefore, of paramount importance in learning to control the mind.

The following analogy will help to make the relationship between *prana* and other aspects of one's being more clear: In the palace of the human body there are seven chambers. The king and queen (the soul and the intellect) are sitting in the first, or innermost, chamber. In the second and third chambers are the offices of the ministers (the mind), some of whom are working by day and others by night. In the fourth chamber is the office of the bodyguard of the king (the chief breath). Ten minor breaths are subordinate guards under him, and they perform their duties at the command of the chief breath. There are three other chambers, and the king, with the help of the officers (the senses and the body), has full authority over them. Here we will discuss the role of the chief breath and its subordinates.

In this government of the human body the breath

plays a very vital role, for it establishes relationships between the mind and body. After working for a certain period of time, it finally ceases, and then the senses and the body are unable to work. Even with the passing away of breath, the occupants of the first and second chambers are not affected in any way, but the workers in the third to seventh chambers are paralyzed. After the breath ceases the inner organization remains intact, for the power of the king would not be diminished if the doorkeepers of the palace were to leave their jobs. So when the breath leaves the body, the link between body and mind is broken; the soul, intellect and unconscious mind find another palace and begin their work anew. By the same token, if the guards in the fourth chamber of the palace run away, the king does not worry about it, for he still functions in his inner chamber.

So the wise man who knows that even after death the soul, intellect and mind remain quite intact does not grieve. One who knows this reality is a true yogi. According to the second chapter of the Gita, the wise man is one who has knowledge of *prana* (here, the word *ashu* has been used for *pranas*), for without the knowledge of *prana*, the knowledge of the scriptures is like mere window-shopping.

Pranayama Exercises

It might surprise the reader to learn that most of the time the right and left nostrils do not work equally well. One of the nostrils is always more congested than the other even though the nasal passages are clean and unobstructed by mucus, and this congestion alternates between the right and left nostrils throughout the day and night. Modern physiology is not aware of this alternate blockage, even though it can be tested by anyone and everyone through observation of his own breathing at different times of the day. According to yoga, this phenomenon is a consequence of the alternation of the flow of subtle energy in the *ida* and *pingala*.

For meditation, it is desirable to have equal activation of these two *nadis*, and there are many techniques for achieving this. There are also various methods for changing the flow of breath from the active to the passive nostril. One of them is to keep the active nostril closed for some time with the fingers; the passive nostril will soon become active. Another is to inhale through the active nostril, close it and exhale through the passive. This process is repeated several times and then reversed. Or one can inhale deeply, close both nostrils with the fingers, hold the breath for as long as is comfortable and then release it. This should be repeated a few times, and is useful, especially, when one has a cold or a headache. Another method of changing the flow of breath is to make a fist, insert it into the armpit opposite the blocked nostril and apply pressure with the arm. In a few seconds the blocked nostril will open. In addition, hot and spicy food has a tendency to increase the temperature of the body and cause an increased flow in the right nostril, and exposing oneself to sudden changes of temperature also changes the breath flow.

Changing the flow of breath can cure headaches, depression and other disorders. When the right nostril is predominant one tends to be more active and restless. Right nostril predominance is also conducive to more assertive, or aggressive, activities. Digestion is aided when the right nostril predominates. When the left nostril is open one is in a more passive and receptive mood. When both nostrils flow evenly one has a devotional attitude and feels a sense of harmony and joy. Having both nostrils open is ideal for meditation.

In addition to the *kriyas* described earlier, there is another simple cleansing exercise which clears the nasal passages of obstructions so that the breath can flow properly. Take a cup of lukewarm salt water and immerse the nose in it, closing one of the nostrils with one of your fingers. Inhale the water until it flows through the open nostril, into the mouth and out. Repeat this with the other nostril. In the beginning this might cause a little discomfort, irritation and sneezing, but one soon gets over it. Do this *kriya* each morning, and with time your nasal passages will be unobstructed and you will be free from colds, catarrh, headaches, and the like.

Let us now consider the simpler exercises of *pranayama* as well as a few more advanced ones. The higher stages of *pranayama* will not, however, be discussed because they involve the techniques of *bandhas* or locks. Besides, the higher techniques must be practiced only under the guidance of a competent teacher, not through descriptions given in books. Otherwise, great physical and mental damage could result.

The following simple breathing exercises may be practiced by everyone without any danger. Through them the capacity of the lungs will be increased, and this in turn will increase one's power of resistance to the modern ills of air pollution and the like. The man who practices deep breathing will remain unaffected in situations where an ordinary man would fail.

Simple Deep Breathing Exercises

After morning ablutions, stand firmly in a calm, quiet and airy place. Exhale through your nostrils, keeping the head, neck and trunk erect. Try to keep the body as motionless as possible except for the motion of the stomach muscles and chest that are involved in deep breathing. Apply the root lock by contracting the sphincter muscles of the rectum and pulling them inwards and upwards. Exhale through the nostrils, smoothly, without any exertion and without any sound. Having exhaled completely, do not pause but start inhaling deeply through the nostrils. Do this about ten times every morning for at least two months. Deep, rhythmic breathing, with inhalations and exhalations of equal duration has been proven beneficial for low blood pressure, insomnia and heart attack. It strengthens the nervous system and leads to voluntary regulation of the respiratory system. This is the secret of a healthy body and a sound mind.

Another simple deep breathing exercise is to lie on the back with the feet a comfortable distance apart and the arms along the sides of the body, palms up. Gently close the eyes and place the hands on the upper abdomen, between the rib cage and the navel, in order to feel the movement of the muscles. Inhale and exhale through the nostrils slowly, smoothly and deeply. There should be no noise, jerks or pauses in the breath. Exaggerating the normal breathing process, consciously pull in the abdominal muscles while exhaling. Aspirants who find difficulty in practicing this diaphragmatic movement may use their hands to gently push in the abdominal muscles when exhaling. When inhaling be aware of the abdominal wall pushing out. There should be a slight movement of the chest. Practice this method of deep breathing three to five minutes a day until you clearly understand the movement of the diaphragm.

Relaxation with Breathing

Relaxation with breathing has been proven useful for nervousness and other diseases. Lie down on your back with a soft pillow under your head. Cover your eyes with a piece of cloth and start exhaling and inhaling slowly and deeply, breathing diaphragmatically. First, relax your limbs physically, and then ask your mind to travel, with a feeling of relaxation, toward your toes. Do this systematically, centering on each set of muscles throughout the body and relaxing them. Start by relaxing your forehead, the facial muscles, neck, shoulders and so on, continuing down until you reach the toes. Then return back to the head, relaxing each set of muscles along the way. Do not allow any other feelings to intrude during this exercise.

Relaxation should not be practiced for more than ten minutes at a time. Too much relaxation can be harmful, for if the muscles are relaxed too long the aspirant may lose control over them. What is more, one should not fall asleep during the relaxation exercises!

After relaxing for five minutes, one can create voluntary tension all over the body and try to maintain the state of tension for at least sixty seconds. Then gradually relax all parts of the body again, systematically, from head to toes. Relax, create voluntary tension, then relax again, exhaling and inhaling slowly and deeply. If one concentrates on the deep and even flow of breath and forms the habit of deep inhalation and exhalation, he will find that he can easily relax. In cases of fatigue, deep breathing with relaxation has been proven very beneficial, but retention of the breath should be avoided. One can even relax at one's office desk for five minutes, refresh himself, and thus increase immensely his capacity for doing work.

Nadi-Shodhana—Channel Purification

This is a breathing exercise which purifies the *nadis*, or subtle energy channels. It should be done at least twice a day—in the morning and in the evening. In the morning *nadi-shodhana* is done in the following manner:

1. Sit in a calm, quiet, airy place in an easy and steady posture.

2. Keep the head, neck and trunk straight and the body still.

3. Bring the right hand up to the nose. The index finger and middle finger should be folded so that the right thumb can be used to close the right nostril and the ring finger can be used to close the left nostril.

4.   Close the right nostril with the right thumb. Exhale completely through the left nostril. The exhalation should be slow, controlled and free from exertion and jerks.

5.   At the end of the exhalation close the left nostril with the ring finger, open the right nostril and inhale slowly and completely. Inhalation and exhalation should be of equal duration.

6.   Repeat this cycle of exhalation with the left nostril and inhalation with the right nostril, two more times.

7.   At the end of the third inhalation through the right nostril, exhale completely through the same nostril, still keeping the left nostril closed with the ring finger.

8.   At the end of the exhalation, close the right nostril with the thumb and inhale through the left nostril.

9.   Repeat the cycle of exhalation through the right nostril and inhalation through the left nostril two more times. This completes the exercise.

10.   To sum up, the exercise consists of:

(a) Three cycles of exhalation through the left nostril and inhalation through the right nostril followed by

(b) Three cycles of exhalation through the right nostril and inhalation through the left nostril.

11. In the evening the exercise consists of:

(a) Three cycles of exhalation through the right nostril and inhalation through the left nostril followed by

(b) Three cycles of exhalation through the left nostril and inhalation through the right nostril.

Be careful to see that inhalation and exhalation are of equal duration and are slow, controlled and free from jerks as well as any sense of exertion. With time, gradual lengthening of the duration of inhalation and exhalation should be attempted.

There are many other types of *pranayama*, each having a specific purpose, and some of these will now be described briefly.

Ujjayi Pranayama

This *pranayama* should be practiced in a stable posture with the head, neck and trunk erect. Exhale completely. Now breathe in slowly and deeply through the nostrils. The incoming air should be felt on the roof of the palate and should make a soft, continuous, sobbing sound. This is achieved by a partial closing of the glottis and is most easily done by mentally repeating Soo . . . ooo during the inbreath. The abdomen should be slightly contracted during the inhalation. Now, without any pause, exhale the air slowly through the nostrils. The outgoing air should also be felt on the roof of the palate and should also be audible. This sound is best achieved by mentally repeating the sound Humm . . . mm during the outbreath. This completes one cycles of *ujjayi pranayama*; it may be repeated for about five minutes. The nasal passages are cleared through this *pranayama*, the nerves are soothed and the mind is calmed.

Kapalabhati Pranayama

In literal translation *kapalabhati* means, "the *pranayama* which makes the skull shine." It is practiced in a stable posture with the head, neck and trunk erect and in one line. The exercise consists of a vigorous, forceful expulsion of breath, using the diaphragm and abdominal muscles, followed by a relaxation of the abdominal muscles resulting in a spontaneous inhalation. This constitutes one cycle. Several cycles are repeated in quick succession. In the beginning one attempts between seven and twenty-one cycles, depending on one's capacity. This exercise cleans the sinuses and respiratory passages as well as stimulates the abdominal muscles and digestive organs.

Bhastrika Pranayama

"*Bhastra*" means bellows, and in this exercise the abdominal muscles move forcefully in and out like a blacksmith's bellows. In this *pranayama* both exhalation and inhalation are vigorous and forceful. Together, they constitute one cycle, and several cycles (between seven and twenty-one) are to be repeated in quick succession. There are three variations of *bhastrika*—front bellows, side-to-side bellows and alternate bellows. The one described above is the front bellows.

In the side-to-side bellows the first burst of exhalation and inhalation is made with the head facing front. Now turn the head fully to the right (in the morning, but to the left in the evening) and repeat the rapid exhalation and inhalation. Now the head is turned back to the front and the exhalation-inhalation is repeated. Then to the left—exhale and inhale with a burst—and back to the front. This is one cycle. It may be repeated between seven and twenty-one times.

In the alternate bellows the rapid exhalation-inhalation is done with one nostril at a time. The thumb of the right hand is used to close the right nostril and the rapid exhalation-inhalation takes place through the left nostril. Then the left nostril is closed with the middle, or ring, finger of the right hand and the rapid exhalation-inhalation takes place through the right nostril. This sequence of left nostril exhalation-inhalation and then right nostril exhalation-inhalation applies to the morning practice. It is reversed (right nostril first and then left nostril) in the evening. The exhalation and inhalation should be vigorous and forceful, using the abdominal muscles and diaphragm, not the chest. The cycle may be repeated about twenty-one times. The benefits of the *bhastrika pranayama* are similar to those of *kapalabhati pranayama*: the forceful exhalation cleans the lungs of the stale residual air which is not removed in normal breathing, the entire respiratory system is purified and internal vigor is aroused.

Rhythmic breathing, breathing with relaxation, and both the *nadi shadhana* and *ujjayi pranayamas* may be practiced by the beginner. Then, but only after some practice, the *kapalabhati* and *bhastrika pranayamas* may be attempted.

The advanced stages of *pranayama* involve retention of the breath, and one can harm himself irreparably if he attempts retention without guidance and without disciplining his diet, sleep and sex. Only a competent teacher can advise one to start practicing retention when he is ready for it. Then, as the student progresses, the duration of inhalation, retention and exhalation is extended. Finally, and only after some mastery has been achieved, retention after exhalation is also attempted.

As can be seen, *pranayama* is a complex and highly developed science. The exercises mentioned above are the fundamental ones which can be practiced by all, but there are many more advanced techniques. The student, when convinced of the value of *pranayama*, is urged to seek a competent *guru* in order to learn the more complex practices which involve *kumbhaka* or breath retention, for through such *pranayama* one achieves perfection in action, speech and thought.

FIVE

A Few Glimpses of Concentration

The mind of the average man is diffuse. He is not able to carry a single train of thought through to its desired conclusion, and his thoughts lack continuity, for his mind is greatly controlled by his body and the external stimuli that he receives in his daily life. In reality, however, the body is only a shadow of the mind. It is a mold prepared by the mind for its own expression. Thus it is as absurd for the body to be in control of the mind as it is for a servant to be in control of his master.

Concentration consists of bringing the scattered mind to a point of focus, for it is only through concentration that the mind can fulfill its real potential. In concentration all mental energies are brought to bear on one object or idea. The mind of the beginner rebels against the effort to concentrate, for the untrained mind finds it difficult to focus its attention consciously on one object or idea for a sustained length of time. When the aspirant tries to slow down his thinking process, for instance, thoughts resist his effort to control them and flit through his mind at a hectic pace. His mind seems never free from thoughts. When one anxiety is removed, another immediately manifests itself, and his mind remains distracted most of the time. Through imagination and fantasy, too, his mind diverts him from the object of concentration.

The real potential and glory of the mind is hidden behind a veil of instincts, impulses, emotions, moods, sentiments, whims and fancies, so in order to understand how the mind is so veiled we must consider what is meant by each of these terms. An instinct, for instance, is an involuntary prompting into action. All human beings and animals in this world have two powerful instincts—self-preservation and reproduction. Hunger arises from the self-preserving instinct, while lust is a manifestation of the reproductive instinct. Then there are three kinds of impulses—impulses of thoughts, speech and action—which are intimately related to the imagination, and which can be controlled by using cultivated reason and will power.

Emotions, moods and sentiments are interconnected, but they have their separate roles in the mental world. An emotion is a combination of thought and desire, for emotions are desires penetrated by, or merged with, thought. Two basic emotions are love and hate, and many other emotions contain elements of these basic emotions. Reverence, for instance, is a compound of respect and love. Of the many possible sentiments, three are the most important—the religious sentiment, the moral sentiment and the aesthetic sentiment, but feelings and sentiments are illusory in nature and are deceptions created by the mind. Moods enslave the mind. In Sanskrit the word for mood is *bhava*, and two important *bhavas* are joy, or exhilaration, and grief, or depression. Normally, the mind is continually jumping from one *bhava* to another, and as a result, these currents and cross-currents do not allow it to think of higher realms of experience. The only truly beneficial mood is the meditative mood, and in this mood concentration comes in a spontaneous, effortless flow. Whims and fancies are present in all human beings, and in extreme cases they lead to eccentricity. Under the influence of a whim, for instance, the mind is trampled underneath, resulting in misery. Fancy is a conception of the intellectual faculty, of a lighter and less imperious cast than imagination. It helps a poet, an artist or a dancer but not a student of yoga when he is trying to concentrate.

Modern science tries to explain the modifications of the mind in a gross manner by attributing emotions, moods and so forth to secretions of the endocrine glands such as the thyroid and parathyroid glands, pineal gland and thymus. When they are absorbed by the blood these secretions, according to modern science, play a vital part in determining the temperament of the individual.

Yoga science, however, has a far more subtle explanation for the mind's restlessness, for it maintains that man can control his emotions through the control of his mind. Yoga science therefore focuses on our knowing, analyzing, training and controlling both the conscious and unconscious minds. For thousands of years yogis have known that the conscious part of the mind though significant in conducting certain important duties in the external world, is only superficial. The unconscious is far more important, for in it lie the motivations behind man's activities. This fact has been recently realized by modern psychology, and research into the unconscious mind is finally under way. But there are many things that are not yet understood.

In yoga science an analogy is used to explain the mind: The mind is like a lake disturbed by the rising waves of thoughts, or *vrittis*. The practice of concentration helps to still the waves, and when the thoughts are stilled the aspirant can see his reflection in the water of the lake and realize his own true nature. Therefore, according to yoga science, man is not restricted to the three states of waking, dreaming and sleeping. There is a fourth state, called *turiya*, the state of the superconscious mind. To achieve it the student of yoga tries to concentrate and bring his mind to a focus, after which he can expand it to the super-conscious state. The purpose of concentration, then, is to wash off all the aspirant's impurities, to gather together the dissipated energies of his mind and to lead his concentrated mind along one channel to the state of superconsciousness.

In everyday life we concentrate in many ways. We concentrate while inserting a thread through the eye of a needle and while driving a car through a busy street. This concentration, however, is called external, for it is something in the external world that holds our attention. Concentration, or *dharana*, as described by Patanjali, is an internal, mental process, not a muscular exercise. It takes place entirely within the field of consciousness and is directed by our will. In other words, through internal concentration the attention of the aspirant is drawn to an object and is held on it through the use of his will power.

Continued attention leads to concentration.

Attention is therefore a preliminary to concentration. There are two kinds—voluntary and involuntary. Voluntary attention is that which is directed toward an object or idea by an effort of the will. It requires will power, determination and mental training. Involuntary attention, on the other hand, is spontaneous. It is a common occurrence and does not demand any practice or will power; it is particularly noticeable among children. Concentration requires voluntary attention.

Some modern teachers formulate and advocate theories which are designed to justify their own ways of teaching, sometimes even saying that meditation is possible without concentration. This is a false claim because concentration itself, in its advanced stage, becomes meditation. If the wandering mind is not brought home, all the so-called "meditational methods" practiced these days will be futile. The aspirant should therefore understand that concentration is absolutely necessary, and he should not be swayed by teachings which suggest that concentration leads to tension.

There are definite techniques and processes which help in training the mind to concentrate. For instance, the student should have a definite time each day for this purpose—morning and evening hours are best. Concentration should also be practiced under favorable circumstances. One should be alone and have determined that he will not be disturbed for a certain length of time. The room should be quiet, clean and airy, without pictures or paintings on the walls. There should be no drafts in the room, the light should not be very bright and the temperature should be

moderate. Concentration should not be practiced immediately after a heavy meal, as it causes discomfort and
drowsiness. A regulated sexual life aids concentration.
In addition, do not try to concentrate when you are
physically or mentally tired and restrict your initial
sessions to about ten minutes.

Concentration is easy when the posture is steady,
when the mind and body are relaxed and when the nerves
have been purified by *pranayama*. It is therefore advisable
to practice some yoga exercises and relaxation first. Deep
breathing, with regulation of the breath, stills the mind.
The postures recommended for meditation in an earlier
chapter are suitable for concentration, or you may sit on a
wooden chair with the head, neck and trunk erect and in
one line, legs planted firmly on the floor and hands on the
thighs. Do not practice concentration in the supine corpse
posture (*shavasana*), as this leads to inertia and, ultimately,
to sleep.

The mind should be untroubled and free. It should
not be occupied by worldly worries and emotional problems. So yoga science includes several methods for
controlling them. The first is to assume an attitude of
detachment. One should gently close the eyes, withdraw
the senses from the external world, and say to oneself,
"Who am I? I am not the body, senses, mind, emotions
and impulses. I am the all-pervading *atman*, or soul. How
can these emotions and impulses disturb me? I am completely detached." With these positive thoughts, the
impulses and emotions in the mind slowly wane.

The second method of calming the mind consists of
trying to be a mere witness to one's mental activity,

observing silently the thought waves arising in the mind. One should not associate himself with the passing thoughts; one should merely watch them flit by. No attempt should be made to use the faculties of discrimination or will, and there should be no struggle for control of the emotions and impulses, but one should note carefully the degree and duration of conflicts of attention. Repeated effort will bear fruit. The initial attempts may be very frustrating; only patience and perseverance will lead to success. However, if the conflicts are insurmountable the practice should be halted and continued at a more suitable time, for there should be no sense of effort involved in any method of concentration. Effort leads to tension, and tension upsets the nervous system and results in serious discomfort.

There are various types of concentration—gross, subtle, outer, inner, objective, subjective and infinite— depending upon the object of concentration. The choice of the object is an important consideration, for if the object of attention is pleasant, it makes the task easier.

In the beginning one should concentrate on external objects such as a point, a candle flame that does not flicker, a photograph of Christ, Krishna, Buddha, or the *guru*. One could also choose a blue, red or yellow flower or one could use a mirror and gaze at the midspace between the eyebrows in the reflection. The gaze should be steady but there should be no strain on the eyes. It should be held for only a minute or two at a time, but this may be repeated two or three times. The early sessions should not last very long. Intensity of concentration is more important than duration of practice. After a while the time span should be slowly increased.

The nasal gaze and frontal gaze are also effective methods for developing concentration. In the nasal gaze the eyes are gently focused on the tip of the nose, whereas in the frontal gaze the space between the eyebrows is the point of concentration. There should be no violent or forceful effort involved in this practice, and the duration of concentration should gradually be increased from half a minute or one minute to half an hour. The method of concentration chosen should be based on one's temperament, but once the method has been chosen the aspirant should practice it faithfully for at least three months. Only then will he begin to see results.

In the types of concentration mentioned so far the eyes are open and focused on an external object. This is called *trakata*. We now come to methods of concentration in which the eyes are closed. Here, three means are used: (1) Concentration on a word or sound, (2) Concentration on breathing, (3) Concentration on a mental image.

1.   Concentration on a word or sound, such as the eternal word OM, creates vibrations and forms a mental image. When this subtle form is established in the mind, the mind becomes steady.

2.   Concentration on exhalation and inhalation while repeating a *mantra*, or eternal word, brings home wandering thoughts.

3.   Concentration on a mental image also makes the mind steady. In the beginning the mental image

chosen should be that of a concrete, simple object such as a small illuminated circle, or a soothing light, and efforts should be made to hold the mental image for as long as possible. Abstract or complicated objects or ideas should not be attempted in the beginning. Other suitable images are the written form of OM, the form of Christ, Krishna, Buddha or the *guru*.

When the eternal word or spiritual object is chosen by the *guru* the aspirant may have "psychic" experiences such as hearing celestial sounds, smelling exquisite fragrances or knowing the future when these techniques of concentration are used. All these experiences are bright milestones on the path of progress. They help inspire the aspirant, but he should not dwell upon them or consider them to be an end in themselves. They are only by-products of the concentration. The only real goal is ultimate truth and realization.

There are more advanced methods of concentration. In one method the *ajna chakra*, located between the eyebrows, is chosen as the object of concentration. This is the seat of the mind in the waking state and is a very important and sensitive center. Light is seen here during concentration, and this particular region of concentration is very suitable for making the mind inwardly directed, one-pointed and steady. Powers of clairvoyance and retrospection also result from this concentration which in Sanskrit, is termed *divya chakshu*, or "the divine eye."

Concentration on the *anahata chakra*, the heart center, is another method which leads to great joy, for the *anahata chakra* is the seat of all emotions and feelings. It is the yogic heart, between the two breasts, not the heart of flesh. Yogis avoid concentration on the lower plexuses.

It is believed that concentrating on the *ajna chakra* brings all other *chakras* under its command, but those who are emotional and sensitive are advised to concentrate on the lotus of the heart (the *anahata chakra*) while those who are intellectual are advised to concentrate on the space between the eyebrows, the *ajna chakra*. Concentration on either stills the mind. Prolonged concentration leads to meditation and thence to the awakening of the *kundalini* and its passage through the *sushumna*. The aspirant then experiences limitless bliss and realizes the ultimate reality. The awakening of the *kundalini* is possible, however, only with the help of a competent *guru*.

There are many other methods of concentration mentioned in the Upanishads and in yogic manuals, but they are often not elaborated upon and are revealed only to initiates by competent *gurus*. Some of these are *bindu-bhedana, madhu vidya*, and *shaktichalana*. *Bindu* means a point or dot, and in *bindu-bhedana* the *bindu* is visualized at the *ajna chakra* as a tiny transparent pearl until the vision is clear. Then the visualized pearl-like *bindu* is moved to the *sahasrara chakra*. In this practice the *bindu* is regarded as the essence of the mind, and the mind is enriched by direct contact with the resulting superconscious state.

Another very advanced method prescribes concentration on the solar breath of the right nostril (associated with thought) as wedded to the lunar breath of the left nostril (associated with feeling). *Jnana*, or knowledge, is the child born of this union. It is also called *sushumna*, or the joyous mind.

Yogic methods for developing concentration are scientific and exact, and in all of them attention and willful withdrawal of attention are brought under conscious control. Then, in the second stage of concentration, voluntary and involuntary movements of the mind are brought under conscious control. This type of concentration is, therefore, quite unlike that which is taught to us by parents and teachers. The methods used in schools and universities are very one-sided, for they relate to the conscious mind alone. The child is taught how to "take off," so to speak, but no one teaches him how to land. The process of thinking without a definite direction and goal dissipates the energy of the mind, and the thinker does not know how to come back to where he started. Such one-sided teaching can be utterly damaging and dangerous.

Therefore, concentration is an aspirant's foremost duty. According to *Adi-Shankara*, the founder of Advaita philosophy, the aspirant's duty consists of two things: controlling the senses and concentrating the mind. Until the thoughts of the aspirant are completely controlled he should strive ceaselessly, concentrating his mind on one truth at a time.

Concentration is in opposition to sensuous desires. When the mind becomes free, or desireless, free from dwelling on sense objects and their enjoyment, the state of *dhyanam*, or meditation, the state referred to as *nididhyasana* by the Vedantins, is achieved. Concentration is therefore the master key which opens the gates of meditation, for prolonged concentration results in meditation. In fact, it is difficult to discern the dividing line between the two.

Without concentration the energy of the mind is dissipated in vague thoughts, worries and fantasies. A disciplined man expresses himself more clearly through concentration; a man of ordinary intellect, with highly developed concentration, is more creative than the highly intellectual man of poor concentration. Through concentration a direct link with the cosmic mind is established so that the mind can attend to several things simultaneously. Concentration is no substitute for labor or action, but it does assist the individual in gaining unique experiences and truths hidden in the deeper recesses of the mind.

Patanjali gave elaborate treatment to the science of concentration, for he realized its utility in calming an agitated mind. Modern scientists now concur with this view and are convinced that only through concentration can one gather together scattered forces and emotions and resolve conflicts. With steady practice the nervous system and the mind are relaxed, and the mind then becomes steady, one-pointed and free from the shackles of desire. The aspirant is thus led, through concentration, to the superconscious state where he experiences the bliss divine.

SIX

Mind and Its Analysis

According to yoga science the brain gets rest during sleep, but not the mind, (the yogi who has controlled his mind derives the joy of rest from meditation), and it is through the mind that the all-pervading *Brahman*, or universal spirit, manifests itself. In *samadhi*, which is, according to raja yoga, the final abode of bliss, the mind goes to its original seat where its presiding deity resides.

The origin of the mind is *atmashakti* (the capacity of the Self); the seat of the mind is the *Brahma-randhra*— the cavity of the brain. In Sanskrit the cosmic mind is called *Hiranyagarbha, Karya-Brahman,* and *Sambhuti.* According to the Gita, the mind is one of the *ashtaprakritis* or eight primary elements, namely, earth, water, fire, air, space, lower mind, intellect and ego. In raja yoga and its philosophical background (which is *Sankhya* philosophy), the term *mahat* denotes the cosmic, or universal, mind, the first principle manifested out of the unmanifested one, *Brahman.* Just as the wheel rests on spokes, and the spokes rest on an axle, so do our minds rest on the cosmic mind, and the cosmic mind rests on *Brahman*. If we think of the cosmic mind as the source of all individual minds, and if we think of it as represented by energy, then all creatures of the world would be like small illumined bulbs, and just as electricity is generated in a powerhouse and flows into bulbs, so power from the cosmic mind flows into individual minds. The cosmic mind is very subtle, and it is in close contact with other minds. In other words, as one's mind evolves one enters into a conscious relationship with other minds. Numerous minds are linked in this way, and this network forms part of *mahat*, the cosmic mind. This is called the *vibhu* theory of raja yoga.

From *mahat* comes *ahamkara*, or ego and from the *sattvik ahamkara*, or pure tranquil ego, comes *manas*, or the lower mind; from the *rajasik ahamkara*, or active ego, come the *indriyas*, the faculties of perception and action; from the *tamasik ahamkara*, or inert ego, come the *tanmatras*, or subtle elements from which arise the gross elements which form this universe. The mind, as understood by yoga psychology, is fourfold. Together, the four aspects of the mind constitute *antah karana*, the inner instrument, which is made up of: *manas*, the lower mind; *buddhi*, the intellect, or faculty of discrimination; *ahamkara*, the ego; *citta*, the mind-stuff. *Manas*, the lower mind, is the link between the senses of perception and action and the *buddhi*, or discriminative faculty, and it also transmits the orders of *buddhi* to the active senses. *Buddhi* is the correlate of the cosmic intelligence (*mahat*) on the plane of the individual. It is both the will and the faculty of discrimination combined. *Buddhi* sorts out the sensory input, and when it arrives at a decision, *ahamkara* steps in and expresses that decision as a thought such as, "I like this ice cream," or "I wonder who he is," and so on. All of this mental activity takes place in the *citta*, or mind-stuff (the canvas on which the mental activities are painted) and it retains the impressions of these activities in the bed of memory. The unconscious is, therefore, a part of *citta*.

Although it is made up of these four aspects, the mind is actually one unit. It is like a tree. The seed is the idea of "I" arising from the ego, the sprout springing up from this seed is *buddhi*, and the branches of the tree are the *sankalpas*, or thoughts and reflections. The mind extends through past, present and future, having various functions, but remaining one. To give an analogy, a person may be a professor at a college, a husband to his wife, a father to his children, and so on. But he is the same person even though he fulfills many functions. So it is with the mind. When it thinks and doubts, it is *manas*; when it wills and discriminates, it is *buddhi*; when it arrogates, it is *ahamkara*; when it stores thoughts of the past and the present, it is *citta*. One beautiful quality of the mind is that when one of its aspects functions, all the others begin to function, too. Another characteristic of the mind is that it always attaches itself to something objective. It cannot stand by itself and function independently. It is always dependent, in one way or another, on a thought form, symbol, idea or image.

There are three bodies which enclose the *atman*, or Self, and which shroud its true glory. The innermost is the *karana sharira*, or seed body. It is with this body that a yogi passes on from one physical body to another, and it is from this body that the other two bodies arise, hence the name "seed," or causal, body. The next body is the *sukshma sharira*, or subtle body, consisting of seventeen *tattvas*, or primary substances. These are: the ten *indriyas* (the five senses of perception—the faculties of sight, hearing, taste, smell and touch as well as the five active faculties of speech, the capacity to hold and grasp, the ability to move, to procreate, and to excrete); the five *tanmatras*, or subtle elements; the *manas*, or lower mind; the *buddhi*, or discriminative faculty. The outermost body is *sthula sharira* or gross, physical body which is linked to the total mind through the *pranas*. At death the physical body dies and the *pranas* dissipate, while the causal body travels to different realms and is subsequently linked with another physical body. Death is the habit of the physical body, but the *atman*, or center of consciousness, is ever existent. When, through meditation, the stage of *samadhi*, or self-realization, is attained, the causal body also drops off, and the *atman* merges in *Brahman*—the drop of water has become one with the mighty ocean.

The soul is the only source of intelligence, and it shines by its own light; the mind and senses derive their activity from it. The soul is the subject, and the mind is its object. According to the Vedas, the most ancient *rishi*, or seer, is the soul who sees through the mind, and it is a cardinal principle of Hindu scriptures that any subject considers its objects to be non-intelligent. Even the ego, then, is non-intelligent because it does not shine by its own light.

Just as the physical body is composed of solid, liquid and gaseous matter, so is the mind, or "subtle body," made up of various subtle vibrations, and just as physical bodies vary from person to person, so also do the subtle bodies of different people. It is also true that every man has a mental world of his own, and there are vast differences between any two minds, for the mind is both the atomic *anu* and the all prevailing *vibhu*, just as in variety is found the beauty of the cosmic mind.

In Sanskrit we refer to *tejas*—the brilliance that emanates from the mind, for the developed minds of yogis have an effulgent aura which can travel and affect those who are prepared to come under its influence in a beneficial manner. That is how telepathy is established between two lovers, or between a yogi and his disciples. That is how a strong mind influences a weak mind. Some people develop a more sensitive and organized thought-force than others, and one who has purified his mind becomes a center of force. That is why weaker minds are unconsciously drawn to purified minds—because they derive peace, power, strength and joy from the greater force coming from that mind. For instance, in yoga, aspirants are benefited more when they are in the presence of their master. Even though the *guru* may not speak a word the student can feel a thrilling sensation and derive new inspiration from his mere presence. For one who has an undeveloped mind it is necessary to surrender to a virtuous and purified mind, for unless one surrenders the higher mind takes some time to influence the lower mind. Fortunate are those who have such opportunities.

The mind is a collection of thoughts and habits. It

is a huge heap of desires gathered from contact with the different forces of the world, for it is the habit of the mind to collect feelings aroused by worldly disturbances. It gathers impressions from ever-changing sources. It is a storehouse of new and old desires. This constant storage and change does not interfere with mental operations, for some of the old desires depart as new arrivals make their abode in the subtle mind, and the mental harmony of thought, feeling and desire is sustained. The mind changes its color and shade every minute, but beliefs, powers of judgment and discrimination change only after some years, because the mind evolves through its experiences slowly.

Who teaches the mind? It is experience. Man corrects his views with the help of new experience and knowledge. He also builds his conscience in this way, for conscience consists of one's own convictions arrived at either instinctively or by reasoning. The conscience of a yogi and the conscience of an ordinary man, for instance, are entirely different, for the conscience of a yogi is like a clean mirror which reflects brilliance.

Sensation, thought and volition are the threefold functions of the mind, and it has three states—active, passive and neutral. It always rejects monotony. Association, continuity and relativity are the three principal laws of the mind, and broadly speaking, there are three aspects of the mind—the conscious or objective mind, the unconscious or subjective mind, and the superconscious mind.

The mind, intellect and understanding are in the subtle body, but they operate through the physical brain.

We will clarify this statement with the simile of the king and his kingdom: Though a king has complete command over his kingdom and has palaces at different places, he has his most splendid palace in the capital. So it is with the mind. Though the mind has all-pervading power in the body, according to the experience of yogis it has three residences during the three states of waking, dreaming and deep sleep. In the waking state the seat of the mind is the *ajna chakra*—which is situated in the space between the eyebrows. This is its most splendid palace. Just notice what you do in deep thought. You place a finger on the chin, turn the neck to the right, gaze toward the space between the eyebrows and begin to ponder the problem at hand. This shows that during the waking period the mind resides in the *ajna chakra*.

The *atman*, or the source of the mind, is pure consciousness, and the mind is illumined by its brilliance. Just as an iron rod in a fire borrows heat and light, so the mind, being an instrument only and non-intelligent, appears intelligent by borrowing light from its source, the *atman*.

The mind can do only one thing at a time, for it is finite. (In Sanskrit the mind is sometimes termed *paricchinna*, or "limited.") It is ever fluctuating, full of impulses, habits and emotions. It is an instrument through which sensations and thoughts arise, but it must be under the control of someone. For instance, if one controls his mind he will know that the thinker is different from the thought. During deep sleep the functioning of the mind is quieted, so the mind is not the source of life and light. It cannot be taken for the pure Self, for it is full of impurities.

It becomes excited during anger, trembles in fear and shrinks in shock. So the mind is not the *atman*. The human soul is also not the director of the mind because we see that ordinary men cannot control their minds. There is someone else in control of the mind, called *manaspati* in Sanskrit, meaning, "lord of the mind," and if one dives deep into the lake of his thinking, he will find that someone silently witnessing the lake and its various waves. The lake is quite different from the *atman*, and the witness is seated quite aloof from both, but as long as the ripples of the mind are not calmed, the *atman* cannot be seen.

Ordinarily, we make a mistake in defining the word, *knowledge*, not realizing that it has four sources: instinct, reason, intuition and super-intuition. An animal is not able to know because it has only physical consciousness. All of its activities are governed by instinct. In a way, however, the work done by them through instinct is more perfect than that of human beings. For instance, if one notices the excellent work done by the birds in building their beautiful nests, he will marvel at instinct.

Next comes reason. Reason is higher than instinct and is found only in human beings. It is developed by strengthening the faculty of discrimination, and the more it is sharpened, the more the intellect gains the power of penetration. Intellect can travel to higher realms if it is purified, trained and cultivated, and through such an intellect come spiritual flashes. For instance, after collecting facts and reasoning from cause to effect as well as from proposition to proof, the intellect can make judgments and take one safely to the gate of intuition.

Intuition is a spiritual experience. The super-sensory

knowledge of intuition is gained through the functioning of the subtle body. It is a higher source of knowledge than intellect, and in intuition there is no reasoning. It is called the *divya drishti*, or "divine sight," for spiritual inspirations from the inner world come through intuition and not through intellect, and it is through intuition that inspiration, revelation and spiritual insight come. Beyond intuition is the knowledge of Self, and this transcends even the subtle body. This knowledge is the highest knowledge of reality.

The physical body is an instrument by which the mind gains experience from the objects of the world through the five organs of perception. All the senses are used as instruments for gaining experience and knowledge, for the mind is the life-instrument of this body and moves all the limbs according to the data it receives through the organs of perception. Just as a garden cannot exist without water, so the body cannot exist without mental actions which the mind performs with great speed. (The gross body, however, remains ignorant of this.) The body is the projection of the mind, and the mind is the subtle form of the body; the mind contemplating the body becomes the body itself, and is then afflicted by it.

Before anything happens in this outer world of ours, something has already happened in the inner world. Before any action is done, it is done by the mind in its mental workshop. Every cell in this body receives an impulse from every thought that enters the mind. When the mind is turned to a particular thought and ponders it for some time a definite vibration is started, and this vibration repeats itself until it eventually becomes a habit because the body follows the mind and imitates it.

The mind is the subtle counterpart of the physical body, and the physical body is the manifestation of the mind, so when the mind becomes tense, the body becomes tense, and when the mind is relaxed, the body is also relaxed. States of mind are very noticeably reflected on the face, for instance, and just as the tongue is the index of the stomach, so the face is the index of the mind. One may foolishly think that he can hide his thoughts, but thoughts, emotions and sentiments produce very noticeable expressions on the face.

There is a mutual relationship between mind and body. The two are intimately connected. The mind acts upon the body, and the body reacts upon the mind. A pure, healthy mind results in a healthy body because thoughts are the primary cause of all the ills of life. Whatever one holds in one's mind will produce an effect in the physical body. Violent fits of temper, for instance, seriously damage the brain cells, inject poisonous chemicals into the blood, produce shocks in the nervous system that suppress secretions of gastric juice, bile and other secretions in the alimentary canal, drain away energy and vitality, and thus induce premature old age and death. But the pains and sufferings of the physical body are actually secondary to the diseases of the mind.

On the other hand, if unwanted and undesirable thoughts are controlled, all diseases will vanish. Therefore the aspirant should keep a strict watch on incoming and outgoing thoughts, emotions and feelings and should accept or reject them according to their effects and consequences. One is able to do this more easily if the mental atmosphere has been favorably prepared through the *yamas* and *niyamas*. With the right mental attitude, the posture being steady and the breathing deep and even, the senses being withdrawn from the distractions outside, the mind's outward activity is checked and it starts traveling inwards. Awareness of the mind's activities and control of these activities through voluntary attention leads to a state of concentration. The mind is now one-pointed, in a state of focus. That which was diffuse is now capable of penetrating the levels of the conscious and unconscious into the expanse of the superconscious. The aspirant is now in the state of meditation.

SEVEN

What is Meditation?

Meditation is not properly understood in the Western world. Some people think of it as merely concentration, others understand it to be silent prayer. In the *Encyclopedia Britannica*, for instance, the word *meditation* has been explained as concentration, but the word *concentration* has not been explained further. Modern dictionaries define meditation variously as follows:

1. Sustained reflection; the turning or revolving of any subject in the mind; close or continued thought.

2. A private devotional act consisting of deliberate reflection upon some spiritual truth or mystery, accompanied by mental prayer and resolutions as to future conduct.

3. A private religious or devotional exercise consisting of a continuous application of the mind to the consideration of some religious or moral truth, or the like, in order to promote holiness or love of God.

None of the above definitions explains the word *meditation* accurately. It is properly defined by the Sankhya school of philosophy as *Dhyanam nirvishayam manah*, which may be translated into English as, "The liberation of the mind from all disturbing and distracting emotions, thoughts and desires."

Typically, our minds are restless and confused. Our attention flits from one thought to another. Through the course of a single day we may experience many unpleasant emotions such as anxiety, depression, disappointment, anger and frustration, and we are pulled here and there by the many desires which we have. We are easily distracted and find it difficult to find a center of equilibrium, and there is scarcely a chance to find rest and renewal.

Very few people know that meditation is a practice which, from the very beginning, helps us to find stability and calmness. We become freed from the restless desires, from the disturbing thoughts which normally come before our minds and from our emotional reactions. As we progress in the practice of meditation we come to find that disturbances are gradually replaced by an ever-increasing sense of peace and happiness. Our mental and emotional environment becomes purified and we experience a sense of inner refreshment and joy.

Through meditation an aspirant's cognition, emotion and volition become unified, and his latent powers are awakened. Only through such a total integration of the mind can one develop a dynamic personality, but all the glorious deeds in human history have been achieved by men of concentrated will power. On the other hand, western psychologists, psychiatrists and physiologists have begun to realize that the human mind is the originator of conflicting urges and emotions as well, and that many diseases have their origin in the unconscious. What they do not yet know is that these conflicts in the mind can be resolved through meditation.

Meditation begins with concentration, for through concentration the mind becomes steady and one-pointed. When concentration leads to the uninterrupted flow of the mind towards one object, this becomes meditation. The mind is then expanded to the higher realms of the superconscious state. Thus, meditation is the process through which mind is first made one-pointed and then expanded to the state of enlightenment. It involves a subtle yet definite conscious effort.

The science of meditation was developed systematically in ancient India during the Upanishadic period. It was elaborated upon later by the seer, Patanjali, and the practices which were developed spread far and wide. A school of meditation was established for instance, by Indian monks in Egypt around the third or fourth century A.D. and in China around 525 A.D. Later, the teachings traveled to Japan. In fact, the word *Zen* is derived from the Sanskrit word *dhyanam* which means meditation. In the Christian tradition a school of meditation was established by St. Anthony, and the methods of meditation were known to saints such as St. Francis and others, but because of fear that it would become the object of religious persecution, the art of meditation remained secretly hidden in the sacred bosoms of a few wise saints.

Over the centuries meditation has developed into a highly evolved and systematic science for expanding consciousness, for in yoga blind faith is always discouraged. Certain practices are described, as are the results that can be achieved through their use, and the aspirant is expected to convince himself of their validity experientially. With this empirical approach, therefore, a person's firsthand experience of a state of consciousness is the proof of its existence. No other proof can be given; indeed, no other proof is necessary.

In his *Yoga Sutras* Patanjali mentions certain powers a yogi may acquire through concentration and meditation. For example, through sustained and prolonged concentration on the hollow of the throat a yogi can transcend hunger and thirst. Such a claim is verified only by practicing the concentration specified.

So yoga is a voyage of discovery, on which one explores his inner self, aided by the directions given to him by the illumined yogis who have trodden the same paths and reached the final goal. Such directions, both general and specific, are given by Patanjali in his *Yoga Sutras* and in other ancient manuals. However, if we are treading a specific path, each one of us must also seek the aid of a *guru*, a spiritual teacher and guide, for a *guru* is that one person in the world who alone holds the key to ultimate truth.

Methods of Meditation

Let us now consider the methods of meditation. Before the aspirant can attain a state of meditation he should have practiced six preliminary steps, and every time he meditates, he should go through them in order to reach a meditative state.

1. The first step is to establish the right mental atmosphere. Being mindful of the *yamas* and *niyamas*, the ten principles of living graciously in the world and of expanding self-awareness, helps the student in composing his mind and establishing harmony within himself. For instance, if he is in an angry mood he tries to wash away his anger by reminding himself of and reiterating the principle of *ahimsa*, or non-harming. Paying mental homage to the *guru*, and to the long line of sages through whom he has received the teaching, also helps in establishing a favorable mental background for meditation.

2. Before the student assumes the meditative posture it is helpful to go through some relaxation exercises practiced in the corpse posture *(shavasana).* Relaxation can be achieved on three levels: relaxation of the nervous system, the internal organs and the mind. Relaxation exercises range from the elementary to the very advanced ones which aim at withdrawing into the subtle body. Relaxation, with deep breathing, proceeds systematically from head to toe, and back upward.

    Relaxation and concentration are intertwined. One cannot concentrate when one is tense, for tension indicates restlessness and disturbance in both the physical body and in the mind. Systematic relaxation, on the other hand, leads the mind towards concentration as it focuses on the various parts of the body, one by one. Each muscle and joint is relaxed completely through this kind of concentration, and it has been used to cure hypertension, migraine headaches and the like. Physical relaxation also leads to calmness of the mind; alpha brain waves predominate in the relaxed state, and in the more advanced relaxation exercises theta waves (which are indicative of concentration and creativity) predominate.

3.   Having tried to relax body, nerves and mind, the aspirant then assumes a meditative posture which is steady and comfortable and which ensures that the head, neck and trunk are erect and in one straight line. The body should be made absolutely motionless, thus bringing under control the *karmendriyas*, or active senses. One will find that, as time goes by, merely sitting motionless in a meditative posture will induce a feeling of peace and joy.

4.   Sitting in a meditative posture, one should then practice some *pranayama* exercises. These involve control of the breath and vital energy, and purify the body and nervous system. Exercises such as *kapalabhati* and *bhastrika* empty the stale air from the lungs, increase the oxygen supply to the body, make the mind alert and free from drowsiness and will, in time, clear up the nasal and respiratory passages. Breathing becomes more deep and even. *Nadi shodhana* strengthens the nervous system, purifies the energy channels, or *nadis*, and clears the mind. Thus the right and left breaths are equalized and breathing becomes deeper and more gentle.

These breathing exercises eventually lead one to the deeper stages of sense withdrawal and concentration.

5.   The fifth step is *pratyahara*—control of the *jnanendriyas*, or senses of perception. Here, one becomes aware of the space immediately around him, withdrawing his awareness from all other times, and experiences the present moment more completely. He tries to be "here and now," and then makes a determination, or *sankalpa*, by mentally reaffirming, "I am not the body, I am not the senses—they are my instruments. I am not the mind. The mind is my subtler instrument. I am the *atman*, the infinite." Every time the mind tries to wander outward, one should gently draw it back inward.

6.   The aspirant then tries to make his mind one-pointed through voluntary attention and concentration. He now becomes aware of his breath and synchronizes it with a *mantram* like *soham*, "I am He." *Soo . . . ooo* is synchronized with the inbreath and *Ham . . . mm* with the outbreath. One concentrates on the breath, beginning in the nostrils and proceeding inward along the lines of energy channels in the nose-bridge, eyebrow center and spine.

Concentration makes the mind one-pointed, and prolonged concentration enables one to go further, piercing the conscious and unconscious, and expanding the mind to the level of the superconscious. Not all methods of concentration will lead to the superconscious, however. Only the methods prescribed by the *guru*, based on his evaluation of the aspirant's capacity and needs, will lead to the superconscious state. One needs the guidance and grace of the *guru*.

Guru and Mantra

The first stage in guidance is initiation into a specific *mantra*, and then the aspirant may be given concentration on a particular sound, light or *chakra*, along with the *mantra*. Through initation into a *chakra*, or center of integration, the spiritual energy of that center can be awakened, and the blocked channels of subtle energy *(nadis)* can be opened. This cannot be accomplished by the aspirant on his own; it is possible only through the initiatory power of a *guru*, who is a channel for the power which flows down the long line of *gurus*, dating back many thousands of years. There are more advanced stages of initiation beyond this, one following the other, until the aspirant reaches full realization of his divine nature through the grace of the *guru*.

There are two Sanskrit words, *dhyana* and *nididhyasana*, both of which are sometimes translated as meditation. There is a difference, however. *Nididhyasana* should be more correctly translated as *reflection and contemplation*, and it is the method used in the monastic tradition of the Vedantists. (Vedanta is one of the seven schools of Indian philosophy.) In this practice a senior monk assigns a novice a certain truth to reflect upon. The truth is usually contained in a brief sentence such as,

"Thou art That," or, "I am Brahman." Starting with linguistic analysis and discursive thinking, the novice continues to reflect upon the truth until the intellect is transcended; the entire energy of thought is thus absorbed into the inner personality, and the novice begins to realize the inner, intuitive aspect of the truth. Such understanding is, in fact, an inner experience of the truth assigned.

Dhyana, or meditation, is, however, a different process. Here a conscious, voluntary attempt is made to still the activity of the conscious mind. Through withdrawal of the senses and concentration, one-pointedness of mind is achieved, and then, like the continuous flow of oil from one vessel to another, concentration flows into meditation. This uninterrupted flow of the mind leads to timelessness, and intuitive knowledge dawns.

The transition from the one-pointedness of the conscious mind to expansion into the superconscious is possible, however, only through the grace of the *guru*, and without such grace the aspirant who, through concentration, stills the conscious mind, becomes aware only of the murky depths of the unconscious. This is a maze of diverse impressions, and one can lose himself in it so that he cannot transcend the unconscious to attain the superconscious state. Occult sciences, black magic, etcetera, are based on this experience of the dark shadows of the unconscious –a state which represents a fall from the conscious to the unconscious rather than an ascent from the conscious into the purity of the superconscious.

Let us consider some of the techniques which, when prescribed by a *guru*, lead to the superconscious experience (but remember that even though they may be mentioned in detail in books, they do not take the aspirant very far unless they are prescribed by the *guru*). In Patanjali's *Yoga Sutras* various methods of meditation are outlined which are to be used according to the capacity and ability of the aspirant; one such method is *mantra* yoga. The word *mantra* means, "That which liberates the mind from all griefs, sorrows and agonies." It is a secret teaching imparted by the *guru* to his disciple when the latter is initiated into the yoga tradition, and it consists of one or more words, chosen by the *guru*, specifically for leading a particular aspirant to the final truth. It is considered to be sacred. Not every word can be a *mantra*, and they are not composed by the *guru*. They have been handed down to him through his tradition, having been revealed to great yogis and seers while they were in a superconscious state. The science of *mantra* is very exact, and very few people know or understand its true significance, but once initiated, the disciple repeats and meditates upon his *mantra* throughout his life, and gradually it will lead him to the state of *samadhi.*

Japa is the act of repeating the *mantra*, and it has to become an essential part of the aspirant's life. Starting with mere repetition of the *mantra*, the disciple is led spontaneously to meditation upon its meaning and then to the realization of the truth it contains. The *mantra* also works on the level of his unconscious mind, controlling his moods and combating and overcoming undesirable emotional states such as anger, greed, lust, sloth and the like. In addition, it purifies his mind, making him capable of the degree of concentration necessary for his subsequent evolution into superconsciousness. The practice of *japa* is found in most religions of the world and is considered to be a form of prayer by those who employ it.

In the scriptures it is said that when the disciple is ready the *guru* appears. He need not be a human being, however. In the Hindu scriptures there are many instances of aspirants having been initiated in their dreams by great saints, and the *mantras* received in such dream experiences are considered to be as sacred as those received in the waking state from a human *guru*. Concentration upon such a dream experience is also one of the methods of meditation, but the aspirant should be careful not to believe that all of his dreams are of divine origin. The truly inspired dream experience brings with it a sense of joyous revelation and is easily distinguished from other dreams.

Meditation upon the Self

The ultimate goal of meditation is to experience the Self, or *atman*. The Self is pure consciousness, and the experience of Self is a state of transcendent knowledge and bliss. It is that state beyond time, space and causation which has been variously called *samadhi, nirvana,* cosmic consciousness and so on. When the mind is completely centered for an extended period of time, when it is not distracted by various thoughts or external objects, we become aware of the essence of our being, the *atman*. Ordinarily awareness is not refined enough to perceive the Self. The mind is preoccupied with more gross perceptions and thoughts, but the practice of concentration and meditation gradually sharpens our perception of the inner workings of the real Self which is hidden within.

Atman in man is covered by three sheaths. The

outermost is the physical sheath, composed of gross matter. Beneath this is the subtle sheath, composed of subtler counterparts of gross matter. The innermost sheath is the causal sheath which has been fashioned out of our actions by the law of karma. In normal waking consciousness all three sheaths intervene between the aspirant and *atman*, but during the dream state the physical sheath is removed, and in the state of dreamless sleep only the causal sheath shrouds *atman*. We are therefore closest to *atman* in the state of dreamless sleep, but no memory of the experience remains when we wake up, for this sheath is difficult to penetrate. This is why one cannot achieve a realization of *atman* merely through dreamless sleep. One of the methods of meditation consists of trying to bring back into the waking state the experience of the state of dreamless sleep, and it involves dwelling upon, and trying to strengthen, the sense of peace that lingers into the waking state after experiencing the dreamless sleep.

In the Upanishads it is stated that the *atman* dwells within the lotus of the heart, but the words *lotus of the heart* do not refer to the heart of flesh, but to the *anahata chakra*. In the *Katha Upanishad* the *atman* is described as a smokeless, pure, illumined flame the size of the thumb in the shrine of the heart, and in their deeper states of meditation yogis experience the lotus of the heart where, bathed in its inner light, they experience divine bliss. One of the more advanced methods of meditation consists of meditation upon the lotus of the heart after one has made his mind steady through concentration. Then withdrawing from the objects of the senses, one enters this shrine of *atman* and, meditating on it, transcends the body and experiences higher knowledge.

When one first begins to concentrate he is faced with all sorts of distractions. Many aspirants grow discouraged, feeling that they were calmer before they started the practice, but this feeling is only a result of experiencing disturbances that have always existed, but of which one was not aware. It is like seeing for the first time all the dust that has been swept under the carpet. This stage is only one of transition; if the aspirant perseveres he will go beyond it and achieve the necessary one-pointedness of mind.

In the practice of concentration the aspirant concerns himself with the external aspects of objects. Then concentration gives way to meditation in which he perceives the innermost nature of the object of concentration. Meditation finally leads to *samadhi*, in which the aspirant achieves oneness with the object of concentration.

In the lower stages of *samadhi*, though perfect concentration has been achieved, the seeds of desire and attachment still remain in a latent state. Liberation from all bondage comes only in the higher stages of *samadhi* when these seeds no longer exist. Then the mind is opened up to receive direct superconscious knowledge which is beyond all perception of the senses and all comprehension of the intellect.

There are three processes that take place in the mind during meditation: contemplation, filling and identification. The aspirant should remember these three word-images before starting his meditation. Contemplate *atman*; fill the mind with *atman*; then you will become identified with *atman*. As you think, so you become. Think you are *atman*, and *atman* you will become.

Meditation through Self-Surrender

There is one method of yoga in which neither postures nor techniques of concentration and meditation are involved. This is self-surrender, the highest of all the yogas, and it is described by Lord Krishna in the eighteenth chapter of the Bhagavad Gita. (Sri Aurobindo and his followers call self-surrender, "Integral Yoga.") According to this method one should surrender the body, mind, intellect and ego entirely to the ultimate reality in order to bring down into one's daily life the peace, purity, truth, consciousness and bliss of the supreme Self.

The qualities of peace and purity are often misunderstood. When we talk of peace, it is not the peace of the tomb to which we refer. Rather, it is a peace which permeates all aspects of life. It fuses our mind, actions and speech, keeping us balanced and harmonized in all aspects of life. It illuminates our life. Its source is not found in temples, churches or mosques, nor is it found in the rigidity of rituals and ceremonies or in the external worship of idols. It resides in the human soul as a manifestation of divine love. Like the quality of peace, that of purity is often misunderstood, too. Purity means to accept no influence other than the influence of the divine. Mere external washing is meant to keep the body pure, but mental purity leads one from intellect to intuition.

Two other qualities of action characterize the life of the aspirant whose method is self-surrender: faithfulness and sincerity. Faithfulness is to admit and to manifest no movement other than that which is prompted and guided by the innermost consciousness. Sincerity requires the lifting of all the movements of mind, body and action to the level of the highest consciousness and realization where there is no individuality, duality or body consciousness. Sincerity is the unification and harmonization of man around that one central will, the divinity through which we speak, hear, think and feel.

. The *atman* is revealed to that fortunate aspirant who surrenders himself without reserve to the divine alone. For him, calmness, wisdom and the seas of *ananda*, or bliss, overflow continuously. Merely wishing for self-surrender will not help. Merely assuming a mental attitude or having a number of inner experiences are not indications of self-surrender. Compelte self-surrender requires a radical and total change in one's life. In this transformation all of our habits and actions should be surrendered and exposed to the divine light, for without complete self-surrender divine wisdom is not possible. For example, consider the life of an unenlightened man. He lives in the world as an animal, expressing only his own mind, action and speech, satisfying only his own wants and desires. An enlightened man, on the other hand, establishes himself in divinity and then brings forward that divinity from the innermost place so that he expresses it through mind, action and speech. This is a sacred process, but it does not require any effort other than self-surrender.

Without complete self-surrender it is quite impossible for the aspirant to get anywhere near his goal, so in the course of this process one has to keep himself open to the call of the divine force and allow that force to work through both his feelings and actions. If one does not

surrender, he is not allowing this force to work through
him. He is imposing conditions upon it. Divine grace and
bliss is ever-present, but we remain sleeping and unpre-
pared to receive it in our daily life. This is the root cause
of our bondage and misery.

In the early stages of practicing self-surrender,
sincere effort is indispensable, for surrender is not a thing
which can be done in a fit of emotion or in a day. The
human ego resists surrender. The mind has its own ideas
and clings to them. The ego holds sway over the unenlightened man, and we live in a world which is ruled by
ego. But unless a man sincerely desires to go beyond the
mire of ego, self-surrender is impossible for him. For
instance, if there is any surrender at all in the early stages
of practice, it is usually of a doubtful nature, with selfish
demands on it. But when spiritual powers awaken true
surrender occurs. A few aspirants do begin with a true
and dynamic will to surrender, it is true. They constantly
dwell in the Self, and having once accepted self-surrender,
they will not question it. By so doing, they no longer
obstruct their own paths.

Surrender is the way of accepting the divine. Surrender means to offer all one has and not to insist on the
primacy of one's own ideas and desires. Surrender empties
the aspirant of ego and then fills him with divine truth.
If he lets his mind take over, however, discussing and
deciding what is to be done, he will be in danger of losing
touch with the divine force. Then the lower energies will
begin to act for themselves, and this will lead to confusion.
A simple offering of the self to the divine, however,
devoid of egoistic motives, brings immediate results.

What is more, during this process the aspirant does not renounce the world and abandon his duties. He lives in the world. But he lives like the lotus which, though rooted in mud and supported by water, blossoms in air and sunlight.

EIGHT

Samadhi

Concentration leads to one-pointedness, prolonged concentration leads to meditation, and through meditation the mind expands into the superconscious state which is called *samadhi* in Patanjali's school of raja yoga. Patanjali, however, warns us that the practice of concentration must be accompanied by non-attachment, for one who tries to concentrate while remaining attached to the things of the world will either fail altogether, or his acquired power of concentration will lead him into great danger because he will use it for selfish ends.

The danger of attachment is exemplified in the technological progress of modern man. Through the study of the objective world he has been able to harness the forces of nature, but his attachment to the world has led him to misuse these forces. Atomic energy could be beneficial to all mankind, provided man developed an attitude of concern for humanity. Instead, it has become a threat to mankind's survival because man lacks the attitude of sympathy toward his fellow men. The threat of nuclear fission lies not in the nature of the atom, but rather in man's attachments.

Non-attachment does not imply renunciation of the world, although many people mistakenly interpret it in this way. It means perfecting the art of living here and now, performing one's duties skillfully, enjoying life and yet remaining above dependencies on, and addictions to, the objects of the world. When this technique is perfected one can live in the world and yet be free. He can use the forces of nature and the objects of the world as tools to further the expansion of consciousness. It is not necessary for anyone to renounce the world in order to attain *samadhi*.

How does one cultivate the attitude of non-attachment? He can start on the practical level of action. He can read about the great sages of any religion, study their lives, learn to love them and then model his life upon their lives. This will lead to non-attachment in that his love for these ideals will begin to develop into love for all humanity. Another method of cultivating non-attachment is to discover Brahman, the central or absolute reality, manifested in the great sages of history. Realizing that these great men are individual projections of Brahman will soon lead to the realization that Brahman is in all of us, and that we are all one.

There are two stages of *samadhi*. In *savikalpa samadhi*, the lower stage, one retains his sense of individuality. The seeker of truth sees the truth, but retains his sense of "I" as being different from the truth realized. He has to go beyond *savikalpa samadhi* to the stage of

nirvikalpa samadhi in which the seeker becomes one with
the One. Here is to be found the union of *atman* with
Brahman. This stage transcends the stage of intense love
and longing for the ideal, for now the seeker merges into
his ideal, and no sense of duality remains.

Only one who is well established in the stage of
nirvikalpa samadhi is an illumined yogi, and only he can
truly guide other aspirants. Such a yogi is beyond the
bondage of space, time and causation, and he is ever free,
for it is possible for him to remain dissolved in *Brahman*
and yet to return to normal consciousness. He has achieved
eternal bliss.

There may seem to be some resemblance between
withdrawal from the external world in deep sleep and the
highest state of *nirvikalpa samadhi*, but there is a vast
difference between them. One is an unconscious state
while the other is the height of consciousness. Suppose
two people go to see a king. One goes and sleeps before the
king while the other remains awake and enjoys the king's
presence. The one who remains awake is like one in the
blissful state of *samadhi*, while the other, being asleep,
remains in the darkness of ignorance. In deep sleep,
although very near to reality, one is not aware of reality.

Even during sleep a yogi remains fully awake to
Brahman and in the waking state he remains as if asleep to
worldly attachments. In this divine union of lover and
beloved, subject and the object are dissolved in an ocean of
supreme love. It is difficult to express the joy of this
superconscious state. Personal experience is the only way
to realize that eternal joy.

The word *samahitam*, which means "the state where

all of one's questions are answered," conveys the experiential quality of the state of *samadhi*. When all the questions are answered and there is no doubt of any sort, then the mind soars high beyond the level of the languages in which it is accustomed to think. *Samadhi* is not on the level of thinking or even feeling and this is why it is also called *bhavatita*, which means, "beyond feelings." The state of *samadhi*, according to Patanjali's system, is considered to be the highest state attainable by yogis.

In other schools the word *samadhi* is not used. The meditative school of Buddhism, for instance, uses the word *nirvana* to describe the highest state of consciousness—through negation one experiences a void which is called *nirvana*. The school of *advaita* philosophy defines something beyond *nirvana*. According to this school, the highest state is called *sakshatkara*, and it is comparable to the state called *samadhi* in Patanjali's system. Here, according to raja yoga, when the individual consciousness expands itself to become universal consciousness, when *jiva* becomes *purusha*, then the word *samadhi* is used. It is a state beyond mind, action and speech. It is the eighth, and final, rung on the yoga ladder and is achieved when the aspirant establishes his practice firmly, is able to continue his meditation for a long time without interruption, yet with full devotion and reverence and when the subtle sense of self-identity vanishes, allowing control of the latent modifications of the mind. Then *samadhi* is attained.

These few practical hints will help you in your practice of meditation.

1. Whatever spiritual method you follow, practice it systematically and regularly. The reward is immense.

2. Laziness or sloth is the greatest enemy. Life is short, time is fleeting and the obstacles are many. Conquer them by sincere effort and prayer. Help comes from a higher level to sincere aspirants.

3. Just as one eats morning, noon, afternoon and night, so also will one have to meditate four times a day if one wants to realize truth quickly. When one meditates one will develop divine virtues, and a spiritual path is constructed in the mind. If one does not practice regularly and becomes lax, the spiritual path will be washed away by a flood of impure thoughts. Regularity in meditation is of paramount importance.

4. Meditation leads one to the gate of intuitive knowledge which is real knowledge. It is a mysterious ladder which takes the aspirant from earth to heaven. Truth is the *atman*, but one cannot realize that truth without meditation. The paths are many, but one should follow only one path and practice only one method. All the different paths meet at the gate of the kingdom of *atman*. Do not condemn anybody's method or religion, but, instead, follow your own. Methods should not change again and again. The fundamentals of all great religions are one and the same.

The mind assumes the form of the objects it cognizes. When the aspirant continuously meditates on the inner *atman*, he reaches the state of *samadhi*, and in this blissful state nothing is seen or heard. There is no body-consciousness. There is only one consciousness, and that is the consciousness of the all-pervading *atman*. This superconscious experience is called *turiya*, or the "fourth state." The first three stages (waking, dreaming and dreamless sleep) are common to everyone, and the fourth is latent in everyone. When a yogi establishes himself in the fourth state he experiences the living reality in his mind, action and speech. Then he realizes, at all times and under all circumstances, that he is identical with existence, knowledge and bliss *(sat, chit* and *ananda)*. Real spiritual life begins after one enters into this state of superconsciousness. It is the state of divine peace.

Samadhi is not a state that can be attained easily, but if one achieves it supramental knowledge, or intuitional knowledge, is experienced—and one who does not possess this cannot understand the true meaning of religion. In this state the senses, mind and intellect cease functioning, and just as a river merges into the ocean, so does the individual soul merge into the supreme soul—and all limitations disappear.

So often beginners are afraid of this union because they think that their individualities might dissolve or be engulfed. Actually, what occurs is not a loss of individuality, but an expansion of individuality. As long as the individual mind functions within the limited realms of individual consciousness one can meditate, but never attain *samadhi*. The deepest state of meditation, however, expands individual consciousness, and when it has been expanded to its fullest capacity, that is called *samadhi*— sometimes called sleepless sleep, the soundless sound, the highest state of peace, or silence. However we may describe it, this is the highest state which a raja yogi can attain while at the same time remaining aware of his attainment.

Many errors, failures and fallacies face the aspirant on this divine journey. One of the greatest of these is laziness. For instance, after a short period of meditation one may feel like sleeping, and further meditation then becomes difficult. This is because one has not yet formed the habit of sitting in a steady posture and meditating on a single object.

During meditation the aspirant may feel that he is rising from his seat. Some may feel that they are flying in the air. Various persons have different experiences, all of which are functions of the mind, and all of which can become obstructions in the path of meditation. To the wise, they give courage for further progress. Some hear melodious sounds and others see light. Some receive spiritual joy, others get both light and joy. These are temporary phases and may encourage those who pass through them. On the other hand there will be those who will not see or experience any such visions. It is of no consequence. All these experiences are hallucinations, delusions and illusory visions. They are not necessary for progress in meditation.

In the beginning the aspirant should avoid the artificial light of this world and try to make his abode in darkness so that he may see the living light within. Often visions do come from the inner world, but they come and go without leaving any permanent impressions on the mind. These are visions which appear from seen, heard or imagined objects. On the other hand, the more one meditates, the more one's intuition is developed, and it is this intuition that becomes his real guide.

The state of *samadhi* is not commonly experienced, but there are various paths described in the Upanishads to attain it: the path of negation, the path of selfless action and the path of devotion. Emotional ecstasy, however, is not *samadhi*. Inspiration does help, but uncontrolled emotion is very dangerous. In other words, inspirations from the *guru* are definitely beneficial, but ecstasy which is full of emotion cannot be called deep meditation.

A simile will give you an idea of *samadhi*. Four aspirants are at the foot of a mountain. They begin their search along different paths, using different methods and they describe the experiences of their journey differently—until they reach the top of the mountain. When they all reach there, they have the same experience. There they agree that they are all at the same place. This experience cannot be shared with unexperienced aspirants. Mere explanation is like the husk of a grain: one does not discover the nourishing properties of the grain's kernel by studying its husk.

The expression, "All roads lead to Rome," is true, but only raja yoga and its methods of training are scientific and thus subject to scientific verification. Raja yoga leads the student to the final state of realization, not by training the intellect alone, but by training the whole man thus making him more useful to himself and to mankind.

Blessed are those who have attained samadhi.
Blessed are those
who are striving to attain it.

Glossary

The Spelling and Pronunciation of Sanskrit Letters and Words

Sanskrit vowels are generally the same pure vowel sounds found in Italian, Spanish, or French. The consonants are generally pronounced as in English.

a	org*a*n, s*u*m
ā	f*a*ther
ai	*ai*sle
au	s*au*erkr*au*t
b	*b*ut
bh	a*bh*or
c	*ch*ur*ch*
ch	chur*chh*ill
d	*d*ough
ḍ	*d*ough (slightly toward the *th* sound of *th*ough)
ḍh	a*dh*ere
dh	a*dh*ere (slightly toward the *theh* sound of brea*the h*ere)
e	pr*ey*
g	*g*o
gh	dog*h*ouse
ḥ	[slight aspiration of preceding vowel]
h	*h*ot
i	*i*t
ī	pol*i*ce
j	*j*ump

jh	lo*dgeh*ouse
k	*k*id
kh	wor*kh*orse
ḷ	no English equivalent; a short vowel pronounced somewhat like the *lry* in reve*lry*
l	*l*ug
ṁ	[resonant nasalization of preceding vowel]
m	*m*ud
ṅ	si*ng*
ṇ	u*n*der
ñ̃	pi*ñ*ata
n	*n*o
o	n*o*
p	*p*ub
ph	u*ph*ill
ṛ	no English equivalent; a simple vowel *r*, such as appears in many Slavonic languages
ṝ	the same pronunciation as *ṛ*, more prolonged
r	*r*um
ś	*sh*awl (pronounced with a slight whistle; German *sp*rechen)
ṣ	*sh*un
s	*s*un
ṭ	*t*omato
t	wa*t*er
ṭh	an*th*ill
th	*Th*ailand
u	p*u*sh
ū	r*u*de
v	*v*odka (midway between *w* and *v*)
y	*y*es

Vowels. Every vowel is either long or short. The dipthongs *e, ai, o,* and *au* are always long; *ḷ* is always short. Long *a, i, u,* and *ṛ* are indicated by a horizontal line over the vowel. The long form of a vowel is pronounced twice as long as the short form.

Consonants. Sanskrit has many aspirated consonants, that is, consonants pronounced with a slight *h* sound: *bh ch ḍh dh gh jh kh ph ṭh th.* These aspirated consonants should be pronounced distinctly. The retroflex consonants, *ḍ ḍh ṇ ṣ ṭ ṭh,* are pronounced with a hitting sound, as the tip of the tongue is curled back to the ridge of the hard palate. The dentals, *d dh n t th,* are pronounced with the tip of the tongue touching the upper teeth.

Accentuation. There is no strong accentuation of syllables. The general rule is to stress the next-to-last syllable of a word, if that is long. A syllable is long if (*a*) it has a long vowel or (*b*) its vowel is followed by more than one consonant. If the next-to-last syllable of a word is short, then the syllable before that receives the stress.

Adi Shankara *(Ādi Śankara)* Literally, "the first Śankara." Also known as Sankaracharya. He was the preeminent exponent of the non-dual (advaita) school of Vedanta philosophy. In his thirty-two years (A.D. 788-820) he walked the length and breadth of India, organizing the monastic orders of swamis and,

through his skill as a debater, reestablishing traditional Hinduism and its formal philosophy at a time
when Buddhism was extremely popular. His com-
mentary on the *Brahma Sutras* is considered a basic
text on non-dual philosophy, and he has also written
commentaries on the major Upanishads and the
Bhagavad Gita as well as scores of devotional hymns.
To this day the heads of the monasteries he established in the north, south, east and west are
considered to be the final authorities in matters of
philosophy and religion, and bear his name.

Advaita   Literally, "non-dual." The word refers to that
school of Vedanta philosophy which stresses the
absolute identity of the individual Self *(atman)*
with the attributeless, non-dual cosmic reality
(Brahman) and the non-reality of the world as it is
ordinarily experienced. It is described in Shankaracharya's commentaries on the *Brahma Sutras* and
the major Upanishads.

Agni   Literally, "fire." *Agni* is a Vedic deity who is the
messenger of the gods, receiving offerings and
transmuting them so they are suitable for consump-
tion by the gods. In this way *agni* is a symbol for
the vital energy within all things which transmutes
and transforms them from within.

Ahamkara *(Ahamkāra)*   Literally, "the I-maker," or ego.
The function of the mind through which pure
spirit *(purusha)* falsely identifies with material and

mental creation in the Sankhya and yoga philosophies.

Ahimsa *(Ahiṃsā)* The first of five moral restraints called *yamas*, which form the first step of the eightfold *(astanga)* yoga. Their purpose is to curtail behavior which is not conducive to spiritual growth. *Ahimsa* means literally, "non-killing," or "non-harming" and denotes nonviolence in thought, word and deed; it leads to cultivation of "an all-encompassing love towards all of creation."

Ajna chakra *(Ājñā cakra)* Literally, "the command center." It is a center of consciousness corresponding to the nasociliary plexus of the physical nervous system, located between the eyebrows. It is called the "command center" because it is the seat of the mind in the waking state and because when this center is developed all the centers below it come under its command. It governs the energy principle of mind, and its power is awakened by the seed syllable *(bija)*, Om. When the *kundalini* force rises through the *sushumna* channel to this center the seeded *(sabija* or *savikalpa) samadhi* is realized. (See also *chakra, kundalini, savikalpa, samadhi* and *sushumna.)*

Akasha *(Ākāśa)* The Sanskrit word for the energy principle of space. It is often translated as sky, or atmosphere, as well as the inner space, the cave of the heart.

Anahata chakra *(Anāhata cakra)* Literally, "the unstruck center." This center of consciousness corresponds to the physical cardiac plexus located in the hollow just beneath the breastbone in the middle of the chest. It governs the energy principle of air, symbolized by offerings of incense, and controls the cognitive sense of touch and the active sense of the genitals. Interpenetrating triangles, like Stars of David, one inside the other, form the diagram of this *chakra*, and its color is said to be smoky gray or green. Its energies are awakened by the seed syllable *(bija), yam.* The chosen deity of one's mantra or the *guru* is meditated upon at this center, which is the center of feeling and emotion. It is a center for concentration on subtle sound vibrations *(nada)*, and it is said that the *atman* itself resides thumb-sized here in "the cave of the heart."

Ananda *(Ānanda)* Perfect joy. One of the three definitions of *Brahman: sat* or pure being, *cit* or pure consciousness, and *ananda* or pure joy.

Antah karana *(Antaḥ karaṇa)* The "inner instrument" of the mind, consisting of: *manas*, or the active mind; *buddhi*, or the rational and intuitive intelligence; *citta*, the mind-stuff and the reservoir or subtle impressions *(samskaras)*; and *ahamkara*, the instrument of identification, the ego, or "I-maker."

Anu *(Aṇu)* The smallest indivisible particle of matter. An atom.

Apah *(Āpaḥ)* Water. The energy principle of fluidity.

Apana *(Apāna)* One of the five functions of the vital energy *(prana)* governing elimination through the exhaling breath, the kidneys, bladder, colon, rectum and genitals.

Aparigraha Literally, "non-possessiveness." The fifth of the series of moral restraints called *yamas* in yoga philosophy. *Aparigraha* cultivates the slackening of attachments to our own possessions so that things at our disposal become tools and not burdens. It is also intended to develop generosity towards those in need.

Ardha-Matsyendrasana Literally, "The Half-Lord-of-the-Fishes-Posture." This is the first in a series of postures that twist the spine laterally.

Asana *(Āsana)* Literally, "sitting," "position," or "posture." The fourth of the eight limbs of raja yoga, which emphasizes attainment of a steady and comfortable posture. It later evolved into the science of physical culture called hatha yoga in which the word means one of the systems of postures.

Asu The pranas.

Astanga *(Aṣṭāṅga)* **Yoga** "The eight limbed yoga" refers to the eight steps of classical raja yoga as they are explained in Patanjali's *Yoga Sutras.* The eight limbs are: *yama*, or moral restraints; *niyama*, or moral practices; *asana*, or posture; *pranayama*, or control of the breath and the *prana; pratyahara*, or withdrawal and control of the senses; *dharana*, or concentration; *dhyana*, or meditation; *samadhi*, or superconscious meditation.

Asteya   Literally, "non-stealing." *Asteya* is the third of the *yamas*. It includes non-misappropriation of money and non-acceptance of unethical gifts, as well as non-stealing, in order to purge the student of desire for others' possessions.

Ashtaprakriti *(Aṣṭaprakrti)*   The eight principles or elements of the material and mental universe in Sankhya philosophy. They are solidity (earth), liquidity (water), heat (fire), gaseousness (air), space, mind, *buddhi* (rational and intuitive intelligence) and ego *(ahamkara)*.

Atman *(Ātman)*   The individual Self which, according to Vedanta philosophy, is identical to the cosmic Self, the absolute reality, *Brahman*. It is identical in some respects to the *purusa*, or pure spirit, of Sankhya and yoga. That pure spirit is said to be shrouded by five sheaths: the physical body, the body of vital energy *(prana)*, the active mental body, the body of knowledge, and the body of perfect joy *(ananda)*. In meditative practice a yogi gradually pierces these sheaths until he reaches his own inner Self, *atman*, in the highest stage of *samadhi*.

Atmashakti *(Ātmaśakti)*   The power and potential of the Self. (See also *shakti.*)

Bandha   Bondage. The absence of spiritual freedom as a result of *avidya* (ignorance). The opposite of spiritual liberation which is the goal of yoga.

Bandhas   "Locks." Certain bodily gestures which establish connections between energy channels *(nadis)* and aid in controlling the flow of vital energy *(prana)* in the practice of *pranayama.*

Bhakti Yoga   The spiritual path in which a devotional relationship is cultivated with a chosen deity. In *bhakti* yoga the energies which are usually dissipated in random emotions are focused on one's chosen deity and so become a force to propel the student in a definite spiritual direction.

Bhastrika *(Bhastrā or Bhastrikā)*   Literally, "the bellows." A breathing exercise in which the abdominal muscles and the diaphragm function like a bellows, with forced inhalation and exhalation of equal length.

Bhava *(Bhāva)*   "Mood." A state of strong emotion. The word is also used to describe higher states of emotional ecstasy in the path of devotion, *bhakti* yoga.

Bhujangasana *(Bhujangāsana)*   The Cobra posture.

Bindu   The point limit of the mind's capacity which is

pierced through in higher states of meditation in order to bring an aspirant to the superconscious state of *samadhi*. This technique is called, "bursting the *bindu*" or, *bindu-bhedana* in Sanskrit.

Brahma *(Brahmā)*   The first member of the Hindu trinity, characterizing the principle of *rajas*, or energy. He is, therefore, the lord of creation and *praja-pati*, the lord of progeny, or lord of creatures.

Brahmacharya *(Brahmacarya)*   Literally, "walking in Brahman." The fourth of the *yamas*, or moral restraints, *brahmacharya* is also described as controlling one's energies and curbing their wastage through the senses by using the senses skillfully and carefully. Since the greatest loss of energy occurs in the act of sex, this term is often used to mean sexual celibacy alone. It is more properly a celibacy of all the senses, cognitive and active.

Brahman   The absolute reality of the universe, the cosmic Self which is described in the Vedanta philosophy as *sat*, pure being, truth and reality; *cit*, pure consciousness; and *ananda*, pure joy. It exists, however, beyond all qualities and attributes, and so the Upanishads teach that the definition most free of error is *"neti, neti,"* "neither this nor that."

Brahma-randhra   Literally, "the hole, or gate, of *Brahman.*" A spiritual center of consciousness on the fontanel through which a yogi leaves his body voluntarily when the usefulness of his physical body is exhausted.

Buddhi   The faculty of discrimination; the intuitive and intellectual intelligence.

Chakra *(Cakra)*   Literally, a "wheel." Cognate to Latin *circus,* English *circle.* The *chakras* are centers of consciousness in the subtle body corresponding to the major nerve plexuses of the gross physical nervous system situated along the spinal cord. Each center controls a certain energy principle. There are seven major centers corresponding to the principles of solidity (earth), liquidity (water), heat (fire), gaseousness (air), space, mind, and the pure consciousness of the Self. These energy principles, in turn, correspond to particular sensations of subtle (non-physical) light and sound, certain geometric patterns which are used to depict the centers (as well as for meditational exercises), and certain *bijas* (seed syllables) or sound vibrations which form the basis for the science of *mantra* (the repetition of which helps to awaken the energy in a particular center).

Chakrasana *(Cakrāsana)*   The Wheel posture.

Citta   The pool of subconscious mind-stuff into which all the impressions gathered by the senses are thrown, as it were, and from the bottom of which they rise to create a constant stream of random thoughts and associations. According to Patanjali, the codifier of yoga philosophy, "Yoga is the cessation of changes and modifications of *citta*" (Patanjali's second *sutra*).

Dhanurasana *(Dhanurāsana)* The Bow posture.

Dharana *(Dhāranā)* Concentration. The process of bringing the mind, whose natural tendency is to jump from object to object, to voluntary, relaxed attention on a single object. It is the sixth of the eight limbs of yoga described in the *Yoga Sutras.*

Dhyana *(Dhyāna)* Meditation. When the mind has become withdrawn from the senses and concentrated, it achieves a steady, natural flow of attention towards one object.

Divya-chaksu *(Divya-caksu)* The "divine eye." The "third eye" which corresponds to the clairvoyant faculty of the fully awakened *ajna chakra* between the two eyebrows.

Divya Drishti *(Divya Drsti)* Divine sight.

Guru According to the oral tradition of yoga, the syllable *gu* signifies darkness, and the syllable *ru* signifies the dispeller, and so the *guru*, or spiritual guide, is the dispeller of the darkness of ignorance. He is one who has tested all methods of yoga and has experienced everything to be experienced on the

the spiritual path so that he may guide a student past illusory experiences and utilize properly the energies which he is attempting to rechannel. The purpose of the *guru*, as an external person, is to lead the student to the inner teacher, his own true Self.

Halasana *(Halāsana)*   The Plow posture.

Hatha Yoga   The science of physical culture which developed out of the third limb of raja yoga, *asana*. It attempts, through postures and cleansing exercises, to prepare the student for higher practices in yoga. It also denotes the first four limbs of raja yoga— *yama, niyama, asana* and *pranayama*, which are known as the external limbs.

Hiranyagarbha   Literally, the "golden womb" or "golden egg." The cosmic mind, regarded as the first and true teacher of yoga.

Ida *(Idā)*   One of the three principle energy channels flowing in the spinal cord. It controls the breath in the left nostril; it is said to be feminine and lunar in nature, inclining the mind towards intuition and creativity, passivity, calmness and sleep. In the word *hatha* it is symbolized by the syllable *tha*. The goal of hatha yoga is to join the two channels, *pingala* and *ida, ha* and *tha*, into the central channel, *sushumna*, where the mind becomes inclined toward stillness, joy and meditation.

Ishwara-pranidhana *(Īśvara-pranidhāna)* The fifth of the five moral practices in the yoga system. It means, literally, "surrender to the Lord," both in a devotional sense and in the sense of surrender to your own true Self. It must become, in practice, learning to see your Self in others and cultivating surrender of ego to that Self.

Jnana *(Jñāna)* **Yoga** Literally, "the discipline of knowledge." Jnana yoga involves cultivation of one's intelligence, starting from the rational intellect and developing towards intuition whose goal is *cit,* or pure consciousness.

Japa Mental repetition of a *mantra*, which gradually awakens the energy vibrations of which the syllables are the gross representation.

Kantha *(Kantha)* A part of the subtle body corresponding to the area of the physical larynx.

Kaivalya Literally, the "isolation" of *purusha*, or pure spirit, from his false identification with *prakriti*, or material nature. It is the final goal of spiritual practice in the Sankhya and yoga philosophies, and it is the subject of the last chapter of the *Yoga Sutras.*

Kapalabhati *(Kapālabhāti)* Literally, the "shining of the skull" or the "shining of the forehead." A breathing technique in which the abdominal muscles and diaphragm make a fast and forceful exhalation followed by a passive inhalation.

Karma Yoga   The "discipline of action" in which selfless action without desire for personal gain is cultivated. In this way one gradually cuts back on the amount of new impressions (the seeds of future action and of rebirth) gathered by the subconscious. One's actions are gradually purified as meditation is slowly brought into active life.

Karya-Brahman *(Kārya-Brahman)*   The cosmic mind. Corresponding to *hiranyagarbha.*

Kumbhaka   The method of retaining the breath in more advanced exercises of *pranayama.* Retention should not be practiced without the guidance of an experienced and qualified teacher.

Kundalini *(Kuṇḍalini)*   Literally, the "coiled one." The concentrated, fundamental life-energy of an individual, symbolized by a coiled serpent sleeping in its latent state in the lowest center of consciousness *(muladhara chakra)* at the base of the spine. The goal of preliminary yoga practice is to awaken this energy and channel it upward through the *sushumna* channel to the highest center, the thousand-petaled lotus. As the energy pierces each center on its journey upwards, it blooms, as it were, and gradually one's whole being is transformed and perfected.

Kundalini *(Kuṇḍalinī)* **Yoga** A system of practices which includes the use of *mantras, yantras* (the diagrammatical counterpart of *mantra* practice), particular postures and gestures *(mudras)*, and breathing exercises to awaken and raise the latent *kundalini* force.

Laya Yoga Literally, the "yoga of absorption." A system of meditational practices in which the awareness of grosser elements is absorbed into finer ones, progressively.

Mahat In Sankhya philosophy this is the first entity to manifest from primordial nature, *prakriti*. It is the cosmic counterpart of the individual *buddhi.*

Manas Active mind. This word is also used loosely as a synonym for the *antah karana.*

Manaspati Literally, the "lord of the mind (manas)." That which controls the mind.

Manipura chakra *(Maṇipūra cakra)* Literally, the "jeweled city." The center of consciousness which corresponds to the solar plexus located in the navel area. This center governs the energy principle of heat and is symbolized by fire. It controls the cognitive sense of sight and the active sense of elimination through the bowels. Its power is awakened by the seed syllable *(bija) ram.* The diagram of the *manipura chakra* is an upward triangle, and it is represented by the color, red.

Mantra A combination of syllables, or words, corresponding to a particular energy vibration. The student, when initiated by a qualified teacher, utilizes the *mantra* as his object for meditation, and as he practices over a period of time it gradually leads his meditation deeper and deeper. It is the condensed essence of all the teaching the *guru* has to give a student, and it is only through his constant practice of *japa* (repetition) within meditation and in his active life that the power of the *mantra* and its essential teaching will gradually unfold (as its latent mental and spiritual energies are released).

Mantra Yoga The set of practices in which particular revealed phrases, words and syllables (and in higher states of meditation vibrations of subtle sound) are utilized as objects of meditation to awaken a student's spiritual potential. The essential technique is *japa*, or mental repetition.

Matsyasana *(Matsyāsana)* The Fish posture.

Mayurasana *(Mayurāsana)* The Peacock posture.

Merudanda *(Merudaṇḍa)* Literally, the "axis of Mt. Meru," or the "Meru pole." Mt. Meru is the axis of the earth, and the *merudanda* is the inner axis corresponding to the physical spinal column along which rises the subtle *sushumna* channel. Through this channel the *kundalini* force rises along the axis to the highest center as consciousness goes "up the mountain," as it were.

Muladhara chakra *(Mūlādhāra cakra)* Literally, the "fundament" or the "root-support center," it corresponds to the sacral, or pelvic, nerve plexus at the base of the physical spine. It is the resting place of the un-activated, "fundamental" life-energy, *kundalini*, symbolized by a coiled and sleeping serpent. Yoga practices attempt to awaken that energy and to raise and purify it gradually until it reaches the highest center of consciousness where self-realization is attained. This center governs the energy principle, earth (solidity), the cognitive sense of smell and the active sense of the feet. It is represented diagrammatically as a square, its color is yellow and its power is awakened by the seed syllable *(bija), lam*. In ritual offerings one would offer fruits or fragrances as symbols of this energy principle.

Nadi *(Nādī)* A channel in the subtle body for the non-physical vital force called *prana* running roughly parallel to the physical nervous system. Yoga texts claim that there are between 72,000 and 325,000 such subtle channels. The three primary ones are *ida, pingala* and *sushumna*, which run along the spinal column and control the flow of breath in the left nostril, the right nostril and both nostrils together.

Nadi Shodhana *(Nāḍi-śodhana)* Literally, "purifying the *nadis*." A breathing exercise that purifies the *nadis* in preparation for the higher practice of *pranayama*. Also known as "channel purification," or "alternate breathing," it attempts to quiet the mind and regulate the breath by establishing a slow, even rhythm, without a pause between inhalation and exhalation.

Nididhyasana *(Nididhyāsana)* Another Sanskrit term for *dhyana*, or meditation. Contemplation in *jnana* yoga. It is one of the four steps in the intellectual process.

Nirvikalpa Samadhi "Samadhi without distinctions" or the *nirbija*, "seedless," *samadhi*. The highest stage of *samadhi* in which there is no "seed," or object of meditation. There are no distinctions between the knower and the known; there is only knowing, *(cit)*, the pure consciousness aspect of *Brahman*.

Niyama "Observances," or "practices." The second limb of the "eight-limbed" system of raja yoga described in the *Yoga Sutras* of Patanjali. While the five *yamas* or moral restraints, gradually curtail habits of behavior which create obstacles to growth, the *niyamas*, also five in number, attempt to cultivate positive habits which are conducive to self-realization. The practices are: 1) Purity of the body and mind *(shaucha)*; 2) Contentment *(santosha)*; 3) Practices to perfect the functioning of body, mind and senses *(tapas)*; 4) Self-study *(svadhyaya)*; 5)

Surrender of the ego to the higher Self *(Ishwara Pranidhana)*. For a more detailed explanation, each *niyama* has been listed separately.

Om   The highest of *mantras*. The sum total of the celestial and cosmic sound principle, it is said to be the mother of all speech. (Say anything with your lips closed and all that comes out is *Om.*) Its three letters, *A, U* and *M*, represent the elements of all trinities as well as the three qualities *(gunas)* of the material and mental creation *(prakriti)*. There is also a silent fourth syllable symbolizing the transcendent "fourth" state of pure spirit, *turiya*, or *samadhi*. A symbol of the highest realization and knowledge, Om precedes and follows all prayers and the recitations of texts in Indian tradition, and it is found in many *mantras*. From Vedic times it has also been known as *Pranava*.

Pada *(Pāda)*   Literally, "foot" or "part." Also, a chapter. This word is used in the names of the four chapters of Patanjali's *Yoga Sutras: "Samadhi-pada,"* the chapter on *samadhi; "Sadhana-pada,"* the chapter concerning methods of practice; *"Vibhuti-pada,"* the chapter on attainments; and *"Kaivalya-pada,"* the chapter on isolation (of pure spirit from material nature).

Padmasana *(Padmāsana)*   The Lotus posture. A sitting posture for breathing exercises and meditation.

Paramātman   The supreme Self which is one with the individual Self *(jivatman)* in the Vedanta philosophy.

Paricchinna   "Cut off" or "limited." It refers to the mind in its ordinary, limited functioning.

Paschimottanāsana   *(Paschimottanasana)*   The Posterior Stretch posture. A head-to-knees posture to stretch the muscles of the back and the back of the legs.

Pingala   *(Pingalā)*   The *nadi*, or energy channel, which is one of the three running parallel to the spinal column. It controls the flow of breath in the right nostril, and when this channel becomes active one's behavior is characterized by rationality, activity and energy. One might also feel an increase in body heat. The effect of this flow of *prana* is said to be solar and masculine; it is the opposite of the left flow, *ida*, which is said to be feminine and lunar.

Prakriti   *(Prakṛti)*   Literally, "that which makes forth." In Sankhya and yoga philosophy it is the material and mental creation with which pure spirit *(purusha)* has falsely identified himself on account of ego, the "I-maker" *(ahamkara)*. The goal of yoga is the isolation *(kaivalya)* of *purusha* from *prakriti*, the identification of pure spirit with itself. *Prakriti* is said to have three attributes *(gunas)*, or tendencies: balance or purity, *(sattva)*; energy *(rajas)*; inertia *(tamas)*. Everything in the material universe is said to be some combination of these three tendencies.

Prana *(Prāṇa)* The vital life force in any living being which exists in a subtle, non-physical form. It flows through a system of energy channels *(nadis)* which make up the subtle body. The different ways that particular flows of energy affect the body have been given special names and are known collectively as the five- (or ten-) fold *pranas: prana, apana, samana, udana* and *vyana.* The flow called *prana* regulates inhalation; *apana,* excretion and exhalation; *samana,* digestion and distribution of nutrients and energy; *udana,* upward movement of *prana* in coughs, sneezes, peristalsis and death; *vyana* pervades the whole skeletal, muscular and nervous structure and controls blood flow, relaxation and tension.

Pranayama *(Prāṇāyāma)* The science of gradually lengthening and controlling the physical breath in order to gain control over the movements of *prana* through the subtle body in higher stages of the practice. It is the fourth of the eight steps of yoga described by Patanjali.

Pratyahara *(Pratyāhāra)* The fifth of the eight limbs of yoga. *Pratyahara* is the withdrawal and control of the senses, and it protects the mind from the distractions that come to the senses.

Prithivi *(Pṛthivī)* Earth.

Purusha *(Puruṣa)* In Sankhya philosophy this is the pure spirit, the indwelling person in everything. It exists in proximity to material and mental creation *(prak-riti)* on account of false identification of the ego. The ultimate aim of yoga practice is to discriminate between the two, to exist in pure spirit alone (isolation, or *kaivalya).*

Rajasik Ahamkara *(Rājasika ahaṃkāra)* Active ego. Ego with the quality of *rajas* or energy.

Raja *(Rāja)* **Yoga** Literally, "the royal path." Raja Yoga is the classical system of yoga philosophy and practice codified by the sage, Patanjali, in the *Yoga Sutras.* It is also known as the eight-limbed *(ashtanga)* yoga because it is divided into eight steps, some of which were elaborated into separate specialized areas of discipline. Hatha yoga, for instance, the science of psycho-physical culture, developed out of the third limb, *asana,* or posture. Raja yoga is also used to signify the last four limbs taken together: *pratyahara,* or control of the senses; *dharana,* or concentration; *dhyana,* or meditation and *samadhi,* or superconscious meditation.

Rishi *(Ṛṣi)* A seer, especially one to whom a *mantra* is revealed.

Sadhana *(Sādhana).* Literally, "accomplishing," or "fulfilling." *Sadhana* is the word for a student's sincere efforts along a particular path of practice towards self-realization. It is the subject for the second chapter of the *Yoga Sutras, "Sadhana-pada."*

Sahasrara *(Sahasrāra)*   The highest center of consciousness, called the "thousand-petaled lotus," which corresponds to the ventricular caivty of the physical brain. When the *kundalini* reaches this center the unseeded *(nirbija) samadhi* without distinctions *(nirvikalpa)* is realized, the *samskaras* or seeds of future actions are burned in the highest knowledge and the aspirant becomes prepared for liberation.

Samadhi *(Samādhi)*   The superconscious state which is the last of the eight limbs of yoga. In *samadhi* of the seeded variety *(sabija* or *savikalpa)*, one's own superconscious mind experiences the object of meditation, the *bija* or seed directly in its true nature. In seedless *samadhi* there is no longer a need for an object of meditation, and one gains the knowledge of his own self and its identity to the cosmic Self *(Brahman)*. There can be no distinction *(vikalpa)* between the knower and the known; there is only perfect knowing. *Samadhi* is the subject of the first chapter of Patanjali's *Yoga Sutras.*

Samana *(Samāna)*   One of the five flows of *prana*. It controls digestion and metabolism and is said to be situated between the heart and the navel.

Sambhuti *(Sambhuti)*   Another term for the cosmic mind.

Sankalpa *(Saṃkalpa)*   "Resolve." The determination to carry something through.

Sankhya *(Sāmkhya)* A system of philosophy based on the duality of material and mental nature *(prakriti)* and pure spirit *(purusha)*, the goal of which is to discriminate between the two aspects in one's own being and attain the isolation of *purusha* or *kaivalya* (existence in pure spirit). It forms the philosophical basis for the practice of yoga. Sankhya was systematized by the sage, Kapila, circa 600 B.C. and it is outlined in a number of texts such as the *Samkhya-karikas.*

Santosha *(Samtosa)* The second of the five *niyamas*, or moral practices, through which one cultivates even-mindedness and contentment (not satisfaction) regardless of one's material situation.

Sarvangasana *(Sarvāṅgāsana)* Literally, the "posture for all limbs." The shoulderstand.

Sat "Pure being." One of the three aspects attributed to the non-dual *Brahman.* (See also *ananda, Brahman* and *cit).*

Sattvik *(Sāttvika)* Possessed of the quality of harmony, purity and balance which is one of the three qualities *(gunas)* of material nature or *prakriti* in the Sankhya philosophy.

Satya The second of the five *yamas*, or moral restraints. It involves truthfulness to oneself and to others.

Savikalpa Samadhi The lower stages of *samadhi* in which the student becomes one with the inner nature of the object or seed *(bija)* of his meditation and experiences it directly. There are eight stages of *savikalpa-samadhi* which are described in the first chapter of Patanjali's *Yoga Sutras.*

Setu-bandhasana The Bridge posture.

Shakti *(Śakti)* Derived from the Sanskrit root *sak*, meaning, "to be capable of"; it means "power," "energy" or force." It usually denotes the active power of some deity or energy principle. For instance, *kundalini* is also called *cit-shakti*, the power of consciousness or the consciousness force.

Shalabhasana *(Śalabhāsana)* The Locust posture.

Shaucha *(Śauca)* The first *niyama*, or moral practice, through which one perfects the process of cleansing and purifying the body, mind and spirit so that all parts of the personality function properly.

Shavasana *(Śavāsana)* The Corpse posture. A posture for relaxation.

Shirshasana *(Śīrsāsana)* The Headstand.

Shiva *(Śiva)* One of the Hindu trinity of the aspects of divinity, corresponding to the three qualities of the manifest universe (gunas). *Shiva* is the third, representing dissolution, or that through which all things return to their essential nature *(tamas).* He also represents the consciousness principle, of which *kundalini*, the *cit-shakti*, is the active power. In the *tantric* system of yoga practice the goal is to raise that vital energy to the highest center of consciousness, the thousand-petaled lotus, so that they may again become one, dissolving, as it were, into the highest realization.

Siddhis "Attainments" or "powers" which appear when one ascends the higher rungs of yoga practice. They are a dangerous temptation and can become obstacles on the path. They are also called *vibhutis* and are discussed in the third chapter of the *Yoga Sutras*, the *"Vibhuti-pada."*

Siddhasana *(Siddhāsana)* The Accomplished posture. A sitting posture used for breathing exercises and meditation.

Sukhasana The Easy posture. A sitting posture used for breathing exercises and meditation.

Sushumna *(Suṣumnā)* The central channel, or *nadi*, for the subtle energy of consciousness *(cit)* and life *(jiva).* One of three channels that flow (approximately) along the spinal column. The goal of preliminary breathing exercises is to open this central channel so that both nostrils are flowing equally, and then the mind enters a joyful state where it tends naturally to meditate.

Sutra *(Sūtra)*   Literally, a "thread," a *sutra* is a brief aphorism of the kind used by Indian philosophers to record the progression of the main ideas (the thread of meaning) of a philosophical system. They are very terse sentences from which all that is unnecessary has been eliminated. The *sutras*, especially those from the oral tradition, cannot be understood without commentaries.

Swadisthana Chakra *(Svādiṣṭhāna Cakra)*   The center of consciousness called, "her own abode," corresponding to the plexus located just above the genital area. The energy principle centered here is liquidity, symbolized in offerings by water. It controls the cognitive sense of taste and the active sense of the hands. Its diagram is a crescent, colored milky-white, and its energies are awakened by the seed syllable *(bija), vam.*

Swadhyaya *(Svādhyāya)*   The fourth of five *niyamas*, or moral practices. Through *svadhyaya* one cultivates self-study. It includes: the study of scripture and spiritual subjects which leads the mind to meditative pursuits; the examinations of one's own actions in life; *japa*, the incessant repetition of one's *mantra*. It becomes, then, the testing of rationally accepted "truths" in experience and the growth of rational intellect towards intuition. (See also jnana yoga).

Swastikasana *(Svastikāsana)*   The Auspicious posture. A sitting posture used for breathing exercises and meditation.

Talu *(Tālu)*   Palatal area of the subtle body corresponding to the base of the physical skull.

Tamasic *(Tāmasika)*   Possessed of the quality of *tamas* or inertia. One of the three qualities of material creation *(prakriti)*.

Tapas *(Tapaḥ)*   Literally "fire" or "heat." The third *niyama*, or moral observance, which includes austerities to perfect the body, mind and senses and to give rise to fervent determination for realization.

Tattva   Literally "that-ness." *Tattva* denotes the distinctive and elemental state of a thing. In Sankhya philosophy the *tattvas* are the evolutes of primal *prakriti*, especially five physical states of matter, (i.e., the solidity of earth, the liquidity of water, the heat of fire, etc.).

Tejas   The brilliance that emanates from the mind.

Turiya   Literally, "the fourth." The superconscious state of *samadhi* which transcends the three states of waking, dreaming and deep sleep.

Trataka *(Trāṭaka)*   The practice of gazing in order to strengthen concentration.

Udana *(Udāna)*   One of the five major flows of *prana*. It controls the region of the body above the larynx and governs our senses (sight, hearing, smell and taste), coughing, sneezing and peristalsis. It is also the instrument of death.

Upanishads *(Upaniṣads)*   The most philosophical portion of the Vedas and the most recent in the series of Vedic texts. The essence of the Vedic teachings is condensed in these writings.

Vayu *(Vāyu)*   Air. The Sanskrit term for the energy principle of air, or gaseousness. The word is also sometimes used for the *pranas*.

Vedantin *(Vedāntin)*   Those who profess the Vedanta philosophy. The word usually refers to the followers of the "non-dual," or Advaita-vedanta who are also called *advaitins.*

Vibhu   Literally, "all-pervading." It is through the realization of the all-pervading nature of the Self that a yogi gains control over his environment and, consequently, what appear to be miraculous powers or *vibhutis.* (See also *siddhi*). The word also refers to a theory which holds that all minds are linked ultimately to a cosmic mind, *hiranyagarbha.*

Vishuddha Chakra *(Viśuddha Cakra)*   Literally, "purified." This center corresponds to the level of the base of the throat, along the spinal column. The principle of space is controlled from this *chakra* which is represented by a circle and the color, blue. It is symbolized in offerings by the opening and closing of flowers. The cognitive sense of hearing and the active sense of the mouth are governed from this center whose power is awakened by the seed syllable *(bija)*, *ham*.

Vrischikasana *(Vrścikāsana)* The Scorpion posture.

Vritti *(Vrtti)* Literally, a "wave," or "modification." The train of thoughts that moves through the mind is spoken of as being made up of *vrttis*, or waves, arising from the deep subconscious reservoir of *citta*, the mindstuff. Yoga is defined in the *Yoga Sutras* as the cessation of these *citta-vrittis*.

Vyana *(Vyāna)* One of the five primary flows of *prana*. *Vyana* pervades the whole skeletal, muscular, nervous and circulatory apparatus of the body and regulates its tension and relaxation.

Yama Literally, "a restraint." In yoga five moral restraints form the first of the eight steps of the royal path, raja yoga. The purpose of these abstentions is to gradually eliminate habits of emotional behavior which are not conducive to spiritual progress so that a student may be at peace with his conscience. The five are: 1) non-violence of thought, word and deed *(ahimsa);* 2) truthfulness and non-lying *(satya);* 3) non-stealing and not coveting others' possessions *(asteya);* 4) non-possessiveness and non-attachment to one's own possessions *(aparigraha)*; 5) celibacy of all the active and cognitive senses and the mind *(brahmacharya)*. (For a more detailed description, each of the *yamas* has been listed separately).

Yoga Mudra   The Symbol of Yoga. A particular posture.

Yoga   The school of Indian philosophy, closely related to as Sankhya, which, in addition to its philosophical tenets, includes a whole system of practices through which philosophical "truths" can be tested in actual experience as the students perfects himself physically, mentally and spiritually. It is a universal, exact science of developing human potential and has evolved over perhaps five thousand years of experimentation by its practitioners. It was first codified by the sage, Patanjali, in his *Yoga Sutras* in about the second century, B.C. The word *yoga* is generated from the Sanskrit root *yuj* which means, "to join or apply." Yoga means *union* as well as the systematic *application* of certain practices with tested and proven effects and benefits. In this sense of *application* yoga also comes to mean *discipline*, as in jnana yoga: the "discipline of knowledge."

Yoga Sutras   A manual of 196 aphorisms devoted to the royal path, raja yoga, composed by the sage, Patanjali, circa 200 B.C. It forms the basic outline from which all systems of yoga philosophy and practice claim their origin.

Swami Rama

Swami Rama was born in 1925 into a learned Brahmin family in the Indian state of Uttar Pradesh. Orphaned in childhood, he was brought up in the cave monasteries of the Himalaya Mountains by a revered yogic sage of Bengal, and was ordained a monk in his early teens. As a young man he was involved in an extended learning journey, studying and living with more than one hundred sages in the solitude of the Himalayas as well as on the plains of India.

From 1939 to 1944 he taught the Upanishads and Buddhist scriptures in various schools and monasteries while studying philosophy and psychology at the universities in Varanasi and Prayag. He earned a medical degree from Darbhanga Homeopathic Medical School in 1945, and then studied Tibetan scriptures in Tibet from 1946 to 1947.

In 1949 Swami Rama became the Shankaracharya of Karvirpitham. This is the highest spiritual post in India, but in 1952 he renounced this high office and dedicated his life to creating a bridge between the East and the West by establishing a center of learning from where the message of the Himalayan sages could be faithfully delivered. He has founded numerous centers of the Himalayan International Institute of Yoga Science and Philosophy in India, Japan, Europe, and the United States. Dedicated to the benefit and edification of all humanity, the Institute offers a wide variety of educational, research, and therapeutic programs.

Swami Rama is the author of many books, including *Living with the Himalayan Masters, Choosing a Path, A Practical Guide to Holistic Health, Book of Wisdom, Freedom from the Bondage of Karma,* and *Inspired Thoughts of Swami Rama.*

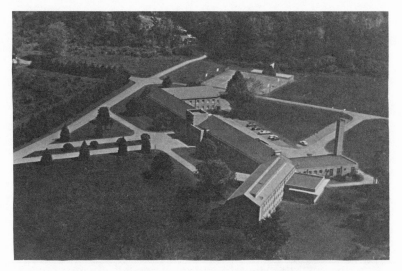

The main building of the national headquarters, Honesdale, Pa.

The Himalayan Institute

The Himalayan International Institute of Yoga Science and Philosophy of the U.S.A. is a nonprofit organization devoted to the scientific and spiritual progress of modern humanity. Founded in 1971 by Sri Swami Rama, the Institute combines Western and Eastern teachings and techniques to develop educational, therapeutic, and research programs for serving people in today's world. The goals of the Institute are to teach meditational techniques for the growth of individuals and their society, to make known the harmonious view of world religions and philosophies, and to undertake scientific research for the benefit of humankind.

This challenging task is met by people of all ages, all walks of life, and all faiths who attend and participate in the Institute courses and seminars. These programs, which are given on a continuing basis, are designed in order that one may discover for oneself how to live more creatively. In the words of Swami Rama, "By being aware of one's own potential and abilities, one can become a perfect citizen, help the nation, and serve humanity."

The Institute has branch centers and affiliates throughout the United States. The 422-acre campus of the national headquarters, located in the Pocono Mountains of northeastern Pennsylvania, serves as the coordination center for all the Institute activities, which include a wide variety of innovative programs in education, research, and therapy, combining Eastern and Western approaches to self-awareness and self-directed change.

SEMINARS, LECTURES, WORKSHOPS, and CLASSES are available throughout the year, providing intensive training and experience in such topics as Superconscious Meditation, hatha yoga, philosophy, psychology, and various aspects of personal growth and holistic health. The *Himalayan News*, a free bimonthly publication, announces the current programs.

The RESIDENTIAL and SELF-TRANSFORMATION PROGRAMS provide training in the basic yoga disciplines— diet, ethical behavior, hatha yoga, and meditation. Students are also given guidance in a philosophy of living in a community environment.

The PROGRAM IN EASTERN STUDIES AND COM-PARATIVE PSYCHOLOGY is the first curriculum offered by an educational institution that provides a systematic synthesis of Western empirical sciences with Eastern introspective sciences using both practical and traditional approaches to education. The University of Scranton, by an agreement of affiliation with the Himalayan Institute, is prepared to grant credits for coursework in this program, and upon successful completion of the program awards a Master of Science degree.

The five-day STRESS MANAGEMENT/PHYSICAL FIT-NESS PROGRAM offers practical and individualized training that can be used to control the stress response. This includes biofeedback, relaxation skills, exercise, diet, breathing techniques, and meditation.

A yearly INTERNATIONAL CONGRESS, sponsored by the Institute, is devoted to the scientific and spiritual progress of modern humanity. Through lectures, workshops, seminars, and practical demonstrations, it provides a forum for professionals and lay people to share their knowledge and research. The ELEANOR N. DANA RESEARCH LABORATORY is the psychophysiological laboratory of the Institute, specializing in research on breathing, meditation, holistic therapies, and stress and relaxed states. The laboratory is fully equipped for exercise stress testing and psychophysiological measurements, including brain waves, patterns of respiration, heart rate changes, and muscle tension. The staff investigates Eastern teachings through studies based on Western experimental techniques.

Himalayan Institute Publications

Living with the Himalayan Masters	Swami Rama
Lectures on Yoga	Swami Rama
A Practical Guide to Holistic Health	Swami Rama
Choosing a Path	Swami Rama
Inspired Thoughts of Swami Rama	Swami Rama
Freedom from the Bondage of Karma	Swami Rama
Book of Wisdom (Ishopanishad)	Swami Rama
Enlightenment Without God	Swami Rama
Life Here and Hereafter	Swami Rama
Marriage, Parenthood, and Enlightenment	Swami Rama
Emotion to Enlightenment	Swami Rama, Swami Ajaya
Science of Breath	Swami Rama, Rudolph Ballentine, M.D., Alan Hymes, M.D.
Yoga and Psychotherapy	Swami Rama, Rudolph Ballentine, M.D., Swami Ajaya
Superconscious Meditation	Usharbudh Arya, D.Litt.
Mantra and Meditation	Usharbudh Arya, D.Litt.
Philosophy of Hatha Yoga	Usharbudh Arya, D.Litt.
Meditation and the Art of Dying	Usharbudh Arya, D.Litt.
God	Usharbudh Arya, D.Litt.
Yoga Psychology	Swami Ajaya, Ph.D.
Foundations of Eastern and Western Psychology	Swami Ajaya (ed.)
Psychology East and West	Swami Ajaya (ed.)
Meditational Therapy	Swami Ajaya (ed.)
Diet and Nutrition	Rudolph Ballentine, M.D.
Joints and Glands Exercises	Rudolph Ballentine, M.D. (ed.)
Theory and Practice of Meditation	Rudolph Ballentine, M.D. (ed.)
Freedom from Stress	Phil Nuernberger, Ph.D.
Science Studies Yoga	James Funderburk, Ph.D.
Homeopathic Remedies	Drs. Anderson, Buegel, Chernin
Hatha Yoga Manual I	Samskrti and Veda
Hatha Yoga Manual II	Samskrti and Judith Franks
Seven Systems of Indian Philosophy	R. Tigunait, Ph.D.
Swami Rama of the Himalayas	L. K. Misra, Ph.D. (ed.)
Philosophy of Death and Dying	M. V. Kamath
Practical Vedanta of Swami Rama Tirtha	Brandt Dayton (ed.)
The Swami and Sam	Brandt Dayton
Psychology of the Beatitudes	Arpita, Ph.D.
Himalayan Mountain Cookery	Martha Ballentine
The Yoga Way Cookbook	Himalayan Institute